"The title says it all! This is a straightforward approach to the paleo concept that will help you look, feel and perform your best."

—Robb Wolf, RobbWolf.com and author of The Paleo Solution: The Original Human Diet

"Alison offers a unique and much-needed tool with *The Modern, No-Nonsense Guide to Paleo*. Having a template to help us live a paleo lifestyle in modern times is necessary as we navigate through our chaotic, stress-filled, and fast-paced world. At every corner turned, we are faced with food temptations, peer pressures, and uncertainties and despite our better intentions, it can be difficult to stay on track with the paleo plan. Fortunately, Alison puts it all in perspective and gives us the tools to stay focused on what matters most; our health!"

—Sarah Fragoso, Everyday Paleo

"I can hold your hand in the kitchen, but Alison's the one who'll keep you on the paleo straight-and-narrow. Her book offers smart strategies and actionable plans to kick start a new, healthy lifestyle – and stick to it."

—Michelle Tam, Nom Nom Paleo

"You've probably heard about the concept of paleo/primal living over the past few years. But you may not have a clue about what it actually takes to implement these healthy lifestyle principles into your modern-day life. That's where Alison Golden swoops in like a superhero to save the day by cutting through the complexities of every aspect of your diet to deliver a walloping blow to the conventional nutritional wisdom that's had us needlessly cutting our fat and consuming more whole grains. Nevermore!"

—Jimmy Moore, Livin' La Vida Low-Carb

"For just one moment, imagine your favorite teacher: the one who was smart, funny, always encouraged you, and made sure you were successful in whatever you did. This is Alison Golden. Her conversational tone puts you at ease – even if you made a mistake (or three) on this paleo journey. *The Modern, No-Nonsense Guide to Paleo* is about more than just "eating paleo". It is a how-to guide in making this a lifestyle. I have been on this journey for two years and yet picked up some great information from this book. This is a great read for anyone from beginner to long-timer."

—Orleatha Smith, Level Health and Nutrition

"As a parent of nine kids that "hang out" with plenty of non-paleo friends, I absolutely love how this book helps parents make practical decisions regarding their own health and the health of their children. Alison's action steps teach beginner and veteran paleo advocates ways that will help them truly become who they want to be as they enjoy the gastronomical experience that paleo has to offer. It's different than any other paleo book I've read and will help you live 'Paleo in a Non-Paleo World'."

—Brad Fackrell, Paleo30DayChallenge.com

"The thing that amazes me most about Alison is she is a true student of paleo and the lifestyle that defines it. She is constantly picking the brains of the best and the brightest to find out what they do, why it works and how that information can be dispensed to those who need it most. This book is a collection of everything she has discovered with one slight twist. It's real and it's practical so people know what they are getting into, and what they need to do to have the success they truly deserve."

—Dean Dwyer, DeanDwyer.com

"This book covers all the basics to educate, motivate and guide everyone to better health. Alison's sincere commitment to supporting the health of others is evident and comes from experience. She understands how difficult it can be to develop and sustain healthy eating habits. What a great resource with all the tools to look and feel better!"

—Teresa Tapp, T-Tapp Workout

"Just because we want to follow a paleo diet, doesn't necessarily make it easy! But Alison Golden has compiled a fantastic list of strategies and suggestions for developing the skills to make paleo sustainable – for you! *The Modern, No-Nonsense Guide to Paleo* will walk you through both transitioning to a paleo diet and sticking with it over the long-haul, with ideas to help you every step of the way – from organizing your kitchen, to getting enough sleep and activity, to handling vacations and non-paleo friends and family members!"

—Sarah Ballantyne, The Paleo Mom

THE MODERN NO-NONSENSE
GUIDE TO PALEO

DEVELOP YOUR SKILLS TO LOSE WEIGHT,
GAIN ENERGY AND TAKE BACK YOUR HEALTH

ALISON GOLDEN

First Published in 2013 by Mesa Verde Publishing

ISBN 10: 0988795507
ISBN 13: 978-0-9887955-0-1

This book is for educational purposes only. It is neither intended nor implied to be a substitute for professional medical advice. The reader should always consult his or her healthcare provider to determine the appropriateness of the information to their own situation or if they have any questions regarding a medical condition or treatment plan.

Design/Layout: Naomi Niles
Editing: Peter Guess
Photography: Maggie Vittori

For more information about *The Modern, No-Nonsense Guide to Paleo*, please visit http://paleononpaleo.com.

For information about quantity discounts or custom publishing inquiries, please contact alison@alisongolden.com.

This book is dedicated to my sons,
Sebastian and Oliver,
for alerting me to that which I needed to know.

"Every time you eat or drink, you are either feeding disease or fighting it."

—HEATHER MORGAN

CONTENTS

SECTION FOUR: LIVING PALEO – UNUSUAL SITUATIONS

SECTION FIVE: INTERACTING IN A NON-PALEO WORLD

SECTION SIX: BUILDING A STRONG PERSONAL PALEO CORE

FOREWORD

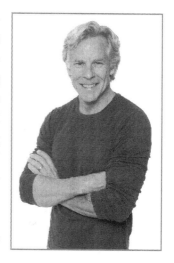

Paleo, Primal, ancestral living, eating, and exercising is taking the world by storm. Mainstream media outlets are pumping out articles about it, new blogs are popping up on a daily basis, and your friends and family are talking about this "caveman diet thing." Whatever you want to call it, ancestral health has officially arrived.

Some people take to paleo like they never knew anything different. It feels natural, easy, right, normal. For these people, going paleo or Primal or adhering to ancestral eating and living and exercising patterns is like going home. Maybe their families support this way of eating, too, making it a simple transition. Maybe they've always kind of eaten this way and giving it a label was just a formality. Maybe they got lucky and never really cared for junk food anyway.

But some people have trouble giving up grains and sugar. Some people don't have the support system to make paleo go swimmingly. Some people need a little extra help, a nudge (or several dozen nudges) in the right direction before taking off. If you're one of those people who want to try eating and living this way, who've had friends and coworkers rave about the massive health benefits they've derived from it but don't quite know where or how to start, this book is for you.

It's for you, because Alison Golden has done most of the prep work. There are lots of paleo/Primal books out there – one in particular is pretty decent, in fact – but Alison cuts through all the extraneous language to focus in on what really matters: concrete steps one can take to go paleo and make it work in a modern world full of tempting junk food, skeptical family members, picky children, life and work-related stress, holiday treats, household budgets, and poor sleep habits.

Beside the intro, there's not really a running narrative that you have to follow. It's the quintessential pick up and read from anywhere type book. You can flip around to various sections depending on what you're looking to get out of it. If you're having a problem with planning bag lunches, there's a section for that. If you need help convincing skeptics, there's a section for that.

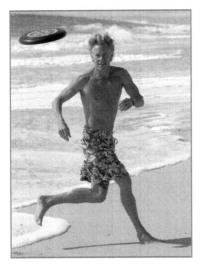

And it's all laid out with actionable steps.

Luckily, this stuff is easy and it is natural – once you get the hang of it and get past the opening night jitters. After all, it's in our genes and our bones and our blood to eat plants and animals, get lots of good sleep, and exercise smartly on a regular basis. The problem most of us have is that we've spent so long divorcing ourselves from this Primal way of life that it takes a little work to get back into it.

The Modern, No-Nonsense Guide to Paleo is one of the best tools I've seen yet to get you started and keep you motivated throughout your paleo journey.

Of course, you're ultimately going to have to do the work yourself. You'll have to cook the meals, buy the food, make the lunches, and fight the temptations . . . but now you know where to begin.

—Mark Sisson

INTRODUCTION

Have you heard about paleo, but it seems too hard? Or you've tried it and feel a failure if you compromise or backslide on following the "perfect" paleo lifestyle? Are you intimidated by the magnificent specimens of health and fitness who bang the paleo drum and feel similar achievements are beyond you?

WHY YOU SHOULD READ THIS BOOK

The principles of the paleo diet and lifestyle are anchored in life encountered millions of years ago. But life today is pretty different from back then, and while much of that is a good thing – nay, a great thing – it can make for difficulties when we want to combine the very, very old with the brand-spanking new.

From the advertisements on television featuring succulent cheese pizza to the grandma at your child's baseball game with her ice cream and cookie snacks, to our societal focus on holidays – so many of them – and our insistence on celebrating with enormous quantities of food, our society is obsessed . . . with eating.

Pivoting ourselves on the axis of life so that we eat as we were meant to – for fuel in order to complete the other tasks of life – is a major challenge under these circumstances. It takes time and effort to uncover the behaviors that have been ingrained in us since birth and perpetuated by those around us. But with continued awareness, practice and sustained effort towards our goals, it can be done, and we can move from erratic, unhelpful and often sabotaging behaviors to a point where our paleo skills are internalized, unconscious and effortless.

With *The Modern, No-Nonsense Guide to Paleo*, you will feel better able to manage this challenge by building the habits, invoking the strategies, and using the tips outlined here. This is the "how of paleo;" how to make better choices, stay consistent, and get healthier, while interacting in a world that not only operates very differently to the way you do, but is also actively pulling you, seducing you, often with care and precision, into its clutches.

WHAT THIS BOOK OFFERS

This isn't a book that covers in detail what paleo is, that's been covered plenty elsewhere. It neither goes into the science to support the lifestyle, nor does this book contain any recipes – there are many others far more talented in those directions than I. Instead, this book is about the skills you'll need to stick with paleo and prevent you from getting sucked into the non-paleo world that surrounds you. In other words, it will help you be successful with paleo in a world that is trying to get you to be anything but. It's full of ideas and processes I've picked up over years of being a life coach, a mom, a productivity and efficiency fanatic and, finally, a paleo advocate.

HOW TO USE THIS BOOK

Each section of this book stands on its own. But like elements of a painting, together they build a portrait. Some strategies work equally well in multiple sections, others are very specific. You can dive right into the section you are interested in, or you can read from front to back (or back to front, if you're wired like that). The choice is yours.

IS IT PRIMAL OR PALEO?

The term "Primal" comes from the wildly successful book *The Primal Blueprint* and is used to describe author Mark Sisson's version of suggested lifestyle practices based upon our ancestral heritage. The main difference between Primal and paleo is that Primal advocates the moderate consumption of dairy products. Please know that when I talk about "paleo" throughout this book, I am using the term interchangeably with "Primal."

 PLEASE GO AHEAD AND WRITE NOTES IN THIS BOOK BECAUSE YOUR ACTIVE ROLE IN CHANGING IS ESSENTIAL. ONE WAY TO DO THAT IS TO SPEND TIME CRAFTING YOUR OWN LIFESTYLE CHANGES. AS YOU GO THROUGH, AND AS INSPIRATION STRIKES YOU, JOT DOWN YOUR IDEAS ON THE NOTES PAGES PROVIDED. KEEP THIS BOOK BY YOUR BED, IN YOUR KITCHEN, YOUR DESK DRAWER, YOUR BAG, OR WHEREVER IS MOST HANDY FOR YOU TO ADD TO YOUR TREASURE TROVE OF STRATEGIES AS YOU GO ABOUT YOUR DAY. IMPLEMENT THESE IDEAS AND REVIEW THEM WHEN THE GOING GETS TOUGH.

SECTION ONE:

UNDERSTANDING PALEO

MY STORY

I first came across the paleo diet back in 2006. It wasn't called "paleo" back then– it was called the "stone age" or "caveman" diet. I found it on some obscure website, the color of which was mostly chocolate brown with an image of Paleolithic man crouched over a fire. It wasn't a particularly attractive look. The website talked about using something called arrowroot and listed a very few number of foods. As our "go-to" food at the time was Mac 'n' cheese out of a box, this alternative seemed seriously extreme, incredibly dull and completely un-doable for a young family. I decided it was only for complete health nuts, and moved on.

I'd been looking for ways to improve my family's health. We were sick a lot, and I was suffering from a whole range of vague, but debilitating health problems. We were spending far too much time at the doctors, and taking too many medications for my liking. I was convinced that our diet lay at the heart of our problems. It had struck me that I had been sick for virtually my whole life. I'd spent much of my early childhood on medications of various kinds. I'd had just about every childhood illness going. I'd had my tonsils removed at age seven due to repeated bouts of tonsillitis. I'd even had scarlet fever. Once my body had dealt with those, my health challenges moved around my body to my skin, my fertility, and a long battle with endometriosis that, although managed with medication, endured for two decades with the only light on the horizon being menopause.

Finally, I devastatingly suffered a second-trimester loss, followed shortly afterward by a diagnosis of Epstein Barr, the virus that causes mononucleosis, from which I just couldn't seem to recover. I'd got to the age of forty-two and could count on one hand the number of years during which I'd enjoyed rude health – and I was so young during those healthy years, I couldn't even remember them! This awareness was eye-opening. Why had I spent most of my years on this earth, sick?

At first, after having dismissed that early version of paleo, I focused on eliminating foods from the diet we typically ate. I removed processed food full of dyes and artificial colors, especially high fructose corn syrup, then salicylates (chemicals found naturally in plants and a major ingredient of aspirin and other pain-relieving medications), gluten and casein. Over the course of four years, I read and tested so many ideas out on my family, they would roll their eyes every time I suggested my latest one. It was only later that I realized I'd been moving in a paleo direction all along without realizing it.

I'd like to say our progress to a clean diet and vibrant health was linear and straightforward, but the fact of the matter was that with little support, our commitment to a healthy diet waxed and waned over those years. We modified our lifestyle, homeschooled one of our boys, and took our own food to parties. But it was difficult to sustain both the kid's enthusiasm and our own for our limited diet. We had seriously different attitudes towards food compared with those of families around us, and I was met with resistance from both within and outside my family. At times, I felt like one of those health nuts I figured must be following that diet I'd rejected earlier!

Meanwhile, we zig-zagged our way through daily life, trying to stay consistent with our diet, but failing many times. I was constantly learning and experimenting. I was gaining skills as a cook, skills that had been non-existent previously, and organizing our meals and our home so that it supported our goals. Each time we fell off the wagon, we'd climb back on again, but I, in particular, was finding it difficult to kick the sugar and wheat products. I had neither a weight problem, nor a health problem that directly correlated with the two foods in my mind, and I resisted enormously the idea they were a serious problem to my health.

I kept resolving over and over to stay away from them. I'd be fine for a few days, but then something would come up, and I'd succumb. Of course, it didn't help that I hoarded both wheat and sugar in their various forms: bars of chocolate, cakes, and packets of cookies were all stashed away in various parts of my house. Doing that made me feel safe. It made me feel I had an outlet for my feelings when things got too much. I could sit down and eat some treat food, and relax. And things did get too much. Daily, in fact. Cakes, cookies and chocolate were my friends, my comfort, and my solace when times got tough. Sometimes, when life was rough with young kids, I felt eating my stash was the only fun I had. I didn't want to give them up. But I was getting increasingly frustrated with my inability to manage my cravings.

Finally, after one vacation back to my home in England, having gorged my way through enough cake and scones to satisfy an army, and frustrated with my seeming inability to resist my treasured childhood foods in even moderate amounts, I resolved that I needed to make some serious changes to my diet. I was still in pain from my endometriosis, I felt exhausted all the time, I couldn't focus, I needed to nap most days, and the anxiety I felt at never knowing if I'd wake up each morning with the energy to complete the day's activity was consuming.

In July 2010, from the moment the airplane wheels hit the tarmac, I stopped eating wheat. That was the only goal I set myself. I had a few failures, but I started to notice the situations that sabotaged me. I would set up strategies ahead of time to deal with them. I made good progress and started to get more confident in my ability to kick the habit.

I was still eating sugar in all its forms, however, and my resolve might have dissolved the way it had in the past if I hadn't stumbled across a reference to paleo by chance on a completely unrelated website shortly thereafter. Cogs started to whirr in my brain, and I remembered the references to it all those years ago. But now things were different. A quick search uncovered wonderfully informative websites, supporting science, and glorious cookbooks!

I grabbed a copy of *The Primal Blueprint* by Mark Sisson, and after reading it, finally felt vindicated. Here was an author stating in black and white what I had intuitively felt for years. Oh, happy day! The support, information, and conviction enabled me to press on, crafting, refining, and polishing strategies, systems and processes to support our conversion to this lifestyle and remove my addiction to sugar. I had learned over the years that it isn't easy to make this kind of change – if it was, we'd all be doing it.

I am now healthier than I have been since I was a young child. My energy is fabulous, and I can focus just fine. I maintain my weight effortlessly. I haven't been sick in months and months. I can go hours without food. I feel proud of my ability to limit the sugar. I can finally live the life I was meant to live.

There is no going back. Now that I've connected the dots between lifelong illness and my diet, and experienced a tremendous improvement in the quality of my life by merely changing what I eat, it's become a no-brainer. But I wouldn't have been able to do that without developing skills in managing the lifestyle and building environmental supports.

Simply knowing what and why we should do something doesn't necessarily make it happen. So, I've put down here in this book all I've learned over the years about the skills involved in embedding paleo as a way of life. Think of it as a manual on the "how of paleo."

Accept only an optimal life for yourself. It's the only one you have. Dream of how you wish your life to be, then put in place the ideas outlined in this book. I wish you great health, much fulfillment and happiness. Enjoy!

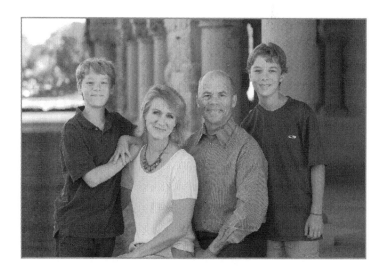

WHAT IS PALEO?

"You can reprogram your genes in the direction of weight loss, health, and longevity by adapting the simple lifestyle practices of our hunter-gatherer ancestors into modern life."
—MARK SISSON, *THE PRIMAL BLUEPRINT*

This is the fundamental principle behind the paleo lifestyle. Paleo means you live in such a way that your body works in concert with your genetic heritage to optimize your health, strength, weight and stress levels. What you eat; and how much you sleep, work, relax and play all fall under the paleo banner as we understand more and more about how our current lifestyle makes us fat, sick, weak and miserable; and how important it is to make a radical change.

DIET

Much of what interests many about paleo is the diet which focuses on the avoidance of foods that have come to characterize our standard twenty-first century diet – grains, sugar, legumes, dairy and processed foods – and instead favors the consumption of meat, fish, fowl, vegetables, fruit, and nuts and seeds along with a good amount of fat.

Eat:	Avoid:
• Meat	• Grains
• Fish	• Sugar
• Fowl	• Legumes (incl.
• Eggs	beans, peanuts
• Vegetables	and peas)
• Fruit	• Dairy
• Nuts	• Processed Foods
• Seeds	• Alcohol
• Healthy Fats	• Starches

These are the basic guidelines. However, opinions vary, and finessing for special circumstances means that one size does not fit all. For example, you'll find evolutionary diet experts advocating the following in varying situations, and with certain limitations:

෴ Dairy consumption

෴ Use of starchy tubers and occasionally rice

෴ Paleo-ish desserts using natural sugars

෴ Consumption of red wine and other alcohol

෴ Different nutritional profiles for women

There is a general 80/20 rule that many follow based on Mark Sisson's suggestion to strive for 100 percent compliance and accept an 80 percent success rate, but others may find this rule to be insufficient to meet their weight-loss and other health goals. Individual experimentation is required to determine this, but the above list is the place to start.

EXERCISE

Being paleo is also about limiting the cardio workouts we have come to accept as essential for weight management and, instead, advocates exercise along lines our ancestors' survival needs demanded. Frequent long, slow walks mimic Paleolithic man's travels in search of food every day; lifting heavy weights align with his efforts to build shelters, make tools, and carry wood and dead animals; and occasional short sprints (without the danger) replicate how he would run to hunt down animals or escape predators.

TIME AND HEALTH ARE TWO PRECIOUS ASSETS THAT WE DON'T RECOGNIZE AND APPRECIATE UNTIL THEY HAVE BEEN DEPLETED.

~ DENIS WAITLEY

This kind of exercising is very different from the hours of cardio-dominant exercise programs we typically do today, and also very different from the primarily sedentary lives we lead. We somehow need to close the gap between chronic cardio and being completely sedentary. Paleo provides the bridge to do this. *Being* paleo, *doing* paleo, and *going* paleo are about **thinking** paleo and making choices that are more congruent with our ancestral heritage than our typical twenty-first-century society norms suggest.

STRESS AND LIFESTYLE

In addition to losing weight, improving our health, and aligning our exercise along ancestral lines, we should also acknowledge that stronger relationships, more relaxation, and greater stress management all have a bearing on our health and, simply, our life fulfillment. The constant challenge is to limit the deleterious effects of life in the twenty-first century while adapting ancient lifestyle principles to modern-day living. If we can do this, we will not only succeed in life, but also perform at levels that are becoming increasingly rare in our modern-day society.

Living paleo in a non-paleo world is rarely easy, but there is no better time in history to live on this earth if we respect and apply this ancient knowledge. We further benefit if we exploit all the opportunities modern life has to offer. We mustn't simply survive; we must thrive. It is within our possibility to do so. It is what our ancestors set us up for.

TO LEARN MORE ABOUT THE "WHAT" AND "WHY" OF PALEO, PLEASE REFER TO THE FURTHER READING SUGGESTIONS FOUND IN THE RESOURCES SECTION AT THE BACK OF THIS BOOK.

MY PALEO PHILOSOPHY

We all have our own personal set of values that determine our decisions and, from those, our actions and our outcomes. Because of that individual set of values, a decision I make will be different from yours in any given circumstance. What is important to me is likely different from that which is important to you.

I come to paleo with my own brand of thinking, and so do you. Living life to the fullest means compromise, trade-offs, plenty of thought, and decision-making. There are many shades of gray.

I want to enjoy optimal health with lots of energy and a feeling of well-being, but sometimes it is more important to strengthen my relationships or save some time, rest a little, or earn some money. This might require me to deviate from making perfect paleo choices. I may choose to do so if, in the long run, I believe that both myself and those who depend on me are better served.

Do you buy prepared vegetables in the supermarket because you eat more of them if they are all ready for you to cook?

Do you let it all hang out on some holidays and get right back on the wagon the next day or next week?

Do you choose to sit at your computer eight hours a day to earn money in order to take your kids to visit their family over the holidays?

Do you occasionally use your microwave to warm up paleo leftovers because otherwise you might have to dash out the door hungry and then be susceptible to the doughnuts in the coffee room when you get to work?

I do all of the above, now and again. These are the types of decisions we have to make, living paleo as we do in a non-paleo world. They are a reality of modern-day paleo living. I say, don't let the perfect be the enemy of the good.

THE COMPROMISE PRINCIPLE

We all make compromises. We have to; it is part of life. We may vary in terms of what, how and why we make them, but we make them. All of us.

So, instead of disputing each other's decisions about the finer points of paleo, focus on your life, your health, and your leadership role. If you don't have any fellow paleos in your life, be the role model you wish you had. You may not realize it, but your influence on those around you is profound – you can change lives, save them even. Seriously.

The key to designing your paleo lifestyle is in understanding your own personal values; the elements and beliefs that drive you forward. Being paleo in a non-paleo world is about making *conscious* decisions every minute of the day and doing so with a full awareness of the consequences of your actions. Accept that your actions and consequences are the result of choices you make, and as such, hold yourself personally responsible for the outcome of those choices. Millions have died over eons to give you this right to freedom. Don't squander their sacrifice.

YOUR PALEO PRESCRIPTION

For some of us, following the basic guidelines of the paleo diet isn't enough. Many of us are highly sensitive to certain foods or are damaged by our years of eating processed and additive-laden packaged food, grains, vegetables oils, and other "foods" making up the diet we typically see today. We react poorly, even when compliant with the paleo diet. We need to go further.

As someone who had been sick most of her life, I can vouch for the fact that turning back the tide after all those years isn't always as straightforward as dropping a few pounds or certain foods from our diet.

When improving your health, whether it be by losing weight, getting your blood sugars down, or improving (a) your asthma, (b) your fertility, or (c) some other chronic illness or condition, the first actions to take are:

- Get enough sleep
- Lower your stress
- Follow the diet

Make sure you are sleeping enough, not over-working or doing too much exercise, and being compliant with the diet. If, after a few months, you are still experiencing issues, you need to start experimenting on yourself.

Occasionally, tracking down the cause of your health problem is like being a detective. Some puzzles are solved fairly simply. But for others, it will take time. No one size fits all.

Experiment with the paleo combo that works for you – your personal paleo prescription.

Maybe you need to cut out more food or certain types of foods. Maybe you need to add supplements. Maybe you need to create your own combination of foods, exercise, stress-relieving techniques, and supplements, and design a custom paleo prescription just for you.

There may be layers to your problem, you may go down a few rabbit holes, and you may need to request the assistance of others in your quest or make some lifestyle changes.

Whatever you do, don't just follow the basic paleo guidelines and give up if it doesn't work right away. It might take years for you to really dial in your diet and work it all out. It took you years to get to this point, so there may not be a quick fix to your problems. You need time to test and review the results of your n=1 experiments.

So, do that, give it time, and be dogged. Success in life is ultimately about persistence.

PALEO SUCCESS: BUILDING SKILLS IN A NON-PALEO WORLD

I mentioned earlier that committing to paleo had occurred after several years of waxing and waning in terms of complying with a healthy diet. Even after embarking on the diet aspects of the lifestyle, I still had my "off" days. But over time, they have become fewer and fewer until, for the most part, I don't even have to think about it.

So, how was I able to steadily change our diet over time to encompass paleo principles when previously I'd been erratic and inconsistent?

THE FOUR KEYS TO PALEO SUCCESS

- Staying focused on the goal
- Building skills
- Course-correcting as necessary
- Practice and persistence

Improving your health by changing what you eat isn't just about learning *why* you should eat differently or *what* you should eat instead, it is also about learning the *skills* necessary to get the job done. Without recognizing this fact, it is difficult to implement the change necessary to live a true paleo lifestyle.

THE FOUR STAGES OF LEARNING

When we learn a new skill, we pass through four stages:

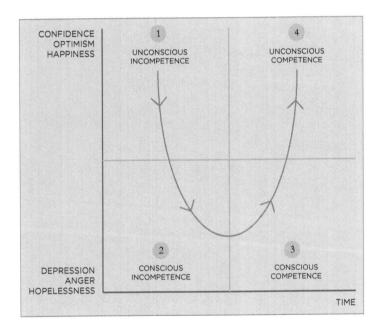

Stage 1: Unconscious Incompetence

This is the "We-don't-know-what-we-don't-know" stage when we lack a certain skill but are blissfully unaware of the deficit or are uninterested in acquiring it. This lack of awareness or disinterest can lead to a confidence that far exceeds our capabilities. As we become aware of the skill and its value to us, our motivation to move out of this stage increases.

Stage 2: Conscious Incompetence

This is the tough stage; it's when we don't possess a certain skill, and we know it. Think of when you first learned to drive a car. You were cranking the gears and over-steering, right? It was acutely embarrassing, most likely. Emotional distress and depression generally accompany this stage, often to the point that we abandon our attempts to learn the desired skill. Intense motivation to attain our goal is necessary to pass through this point.

Stage 3: Conscious Competence

Here, we're starting to learn the skill. We start to transition the odd gear smoothly, we're getting our steering on target, but we're having to concentrate and think about it, often very carefully. Our mood improves, however, often steeply, as we start to acquire the skills. We start to "get it."

Stage 4: Unconscious Competence

This is when we can perform a skill without thinking about every step. Often we're thinking about other things while we're performing them. The skill is integrated and internalized, and conscious thought is no longer necessary. Confidence is at its peak, and your performance of the skill is habitual.

THE FOUR STAGES OF LEARNING *PALEO*

This learning theory describes succinctly the process we go through when we move from being unaware of the connection between our lifestyle and the quality of our health through to achieving mastery with paleo.

Stage 1: Unconscious Incompetence

This occurs when we're young, uninformed, or in denial about the fact that our diet drives our health. We either don't know this connection exists or that our poor health can be reversed, or we don't have any feedback in the form of health issues. Therefore, we can't see the value in eating differently.

Stage 2: Conscious Incompetence

Here, we embark on practicing the tenets of the lifestyle – we resolve to work out more, eat less and better, we go to bed earlier, and we play more often. And while it may go well for a while, we inevitably (because we live in a non-paleo world) come up against a hurdle – a holiday meal, a hard day at work, or a sleepless night with a sick child – and we find ourselves committing a "paleo faileo" and shoveling chocolate into our mouths, buying a ready-made meal, or skipping a workout. When we do this, we're seeking to relieve our uncomfortable feelings. This, though, may cause a vicious cycle to ensue as we beat ourselves up for our perceived failures and turn yet again to our food in a cycle that is hard to stall. Many people bail from paleo at this point, convinced that it is too hard.

Stage 3: Conscious Competence

This is when we start to see successes. Not just those we storm through using willpower, but also ones where we face a challenge to our paleo ways and head them off using strategies we've devised. We're not eating cookies, because we haven't bought any; we've said, "No, thank you" to our co-workers' break-room doughnuts; or we've bought a kettlebell and placed it in plain sight to overcome the inertia that settles when getting a workout requires a drive to the gym.

Stage 4: Unconscious Competence

Everything is dialed in. You can look at cupcakes and not be tempted. Your workout is built into your daily schedule and is as habitual as cleaning your teeth. Your bedtime is 10 p.m. sharp, and your favorite TV programs are on "record." You've renegotiated your working hours to avoid the daily commute. Or perhaps you've moved to a different state or country to reap the benefits of a warmer climate or greater opportunities to support your goals.

Paleo life will always be a work in progress; paleo perfection is a myth. But, with effort, persistence, and an emphasis on the Four Keys to Paleo Success and an understanding of the Four Stages of Learning, we can transition from incompetence to mastery.

THE MYTH OF WILLPOWER AND THE EFFECTS OF STRESS

When we are attempting to achieve anything worthwhile, we need more self-discipline and less impulsivity. As Steven Pressfield says in *The War of Art*, we don't feel any resistance to giving up working with Mother Teresa to work in marketing . . .

When someone starts the process of transitioning to a paleo lifestyle, they typically read up on it, find out what foods they can eat, sign up for a gym membership or other workout program, and off they go, determined this time it will be different. When they stumble, have a paleo faileo, or fall off the wagon, they often give up. If they don't give up, they resolve to do better, pick themselves up, and start over. In other words, they rely on willpower to get them through.

Willpower or self-control is highly desirable. It is something we all want more of – success in life rarely visits the impulsive, devil-may-care types. The famous Stanford marshmallow study[1] and subsequent follow-ups showed clearly that those who exercise self-discipline, even in childhood, are considered more competent and perform better years later.

Willpower is used for self-control, resisting urges, planning our reactions, and careful execution. It is called the pause-and-plan response and helps us resist temptation and override impulses. And it is in direct opposition to our fight-or-flight stress response.

In her book, *The Willpower Instinct: How Self-Control Works, Why It Matters, and What You Can Do To Get More of It*, author

---

1   In the "Stanford Marshmallow Study" of 1972, children were offered one marshmallow. If children resisted eating the marshmallow, they were promised two marshmallows instead of one. Follow-up studies showed that those children who demonstrated self-control under these conditions were more competent and had higher SAT scores more than ten years later. Delaying self-gratification in pursuit of goals was also found to be a life-long characteristic and was related to pre-frontal cortex differences between the two groups.

Kelly McGonigal, Ph.D., writes about how the biology of the body's stress response and that of willpower are mutually exclusive. The adrenaline rush of the fight-or-flight response causes the brain to react instinctively, stealing energy away from parts of the brain that are designed for wise decision-making. Stress will also cause us to focus on short-term goals and decisions while the pause-and-plan response of the brain reflects on the bigger picture. Stress is the antithesis of willpower.

The problem is further compounded when you consider that we have a finite capacity for willpower[2]. Willpower gets used up over the course of a day, even by unrelated tasks. So, the control you showed when you got cut off by that idiot driver this morning during your daily commute may have a direct impact on your ability to resist chocolate candy during your evening. I'm sure you can relate to the effects of a stressful day on your eating habits. Stress and willpower cannot co-exist once a certain level of daily challenge is reached.

 WILLPOWER IS A MIND-BODY RESPONSE, NOT A CHARACTER TRAIT, SO LET THAT ONE GO . . .

---

2   A 2007 study shows that self-control is an important key to success in life and appears to be a limited resource. Just as a muscle gets tired from exertion, acts of self-control cause short-term reductions in subsequent self-control, even on unrelated tasks. Research has supported the strength model with respect to eating, drinking, spending, sexuality, intelligent thought, making choices, and interpersonal behavior. Motivational or framing factors can temporarily overcome the problem. "The strength model of self-control". Baumeister, Roy F.; Vohs, Kathleen D.; Tice, Dianne M.

However, we are not doomed to fail. We can increase the amount of willpower available to us, even if we've been lacking up until now. We can:

- Build up our willpower muscle
- Lower the amount of stress stimulus in our life
- Create an environment that supports the achievement of our goals
- Take up specific habits that increase our ability to pause-and-plan

STRENGTHENING YOUR WILLPOWER MUSCLE

PERFECTION IS IMPOSSIBLE. HOWEVER STRIVING FOR PERFECTION IS NOT. DO THE BEST YOU CAN UNDER THE CONDITIONS THAT EXIST. THAT IS WHAT COUNTS.

~JOHN WOODEN

Your willpower can get worn down, as I'm sure you've seen in your daily life. We resist, resist, resist, and then bam! All your resolve goes out the window and you eat, maybe gorge, your way through the holidays, your vacation, your weekend, or just a bag of chips. Living with a non-paleo person or people can be particularly trying under these circumstances. At times, it feels like that packet of cookies must have a personal line to your brain.

But you can weaken the connection between you and your temptation. Each time you say "No," you are strengthening your "willpower muscle." By training this muscle, with practice and over time, new behaviors become habits, cravings and temptations become less overwhelming, and willpower challenges may even become fun, as shown by those people who take up exercise and end up running marathons! And "No" doesn't have to be literal. Anytime you choose health over disease, you are saying, "No."

REDUCING STRESS AND BUILDING SUPPORTS

All of us, at one time or another, have to up our game to deal with an emergency – a real one or a modern-day crisis such as a major deadline or our boss yelling at us. But some people live their entire lives in situations most of us would consider ongoing high-alert. I know they do, because they write to me and ask me for advice.

It is almost impossible to stay paleo under these circumstances. As we've seen, when we're under stress, adrenaline causes us to make urgent, instinctive decisions that meet the immediate need. Stress doesn't care about our health down the road. Ongoing high levels of stress will sabotage your paleo efforts. It takes time and focus to start and maintain a paleo lifestyle, and if you are being pulled in many directions, that focus will be lost.

If you are experiencing continual high stress over a long period of time, you need to take steps to remove as many of your stressors as possible. Major life issues include high-stress work situations, parenting young children, full-time study, managing a health crisis, moving house, dealing with the death of a loved one, and divorce or a major breakup. These things drain us. Dealing with two of them at once is probably as much as most of us can handle while still maintaining our paleo goals. This is particularly so if you are not completely immersed in paleo life (you live, work, and play among other non-paleo people almost entirely), or you are not yet at the stage where paleo skills are automatic. Recognize the sources of stress in your life; don't blow them off. Cut back on your stress if you are overloaded and build stress reduction into your daily routine.

But often stress is about having too much to do and too much chaos – things could be changed with some paring down and adjustments. If this is the case for you, and you are being derailed, maybe often, there are many things you can do to help support your transition to a paleo lifestyle.

One of themes of this book is that small changes can lead to big results. We can increase our ability to slow down, instill habits that support our goals, and remove behaviors that sabotage our achievement of them. This book is designed to help you do that. It will give you ideas to insert a pause or put an obstacle in your way to allow the decision-making part of your brain to take control and to give you the opportunity to learn new habits by creating a supportive environment in which to do so.

If we don't put these structural supports in place to underpin our efforts, we will continue to fail to the point where we give up. If you are out of willpower by 10 a.m. and reaching for the chocolate, know that there is too much stress and not enough calm in your life. Remember, willpower is not a personal virtue.

NOTES

(BECAUSE YOUR ACTIVE PARTICIPATION
WILL CREATE CHANGE.)

SECTION TWO:
BEGINNING PALEO

GETTING STARTED

So, you've decided to give it a go. Are you ready to jump in with two feet, whole hog, and a part share of beef? Or are you more likely to dip your toe in, try a new recipe, and buy a few extra cuts of meat until you're sure? Okay, I'm mixing my metaphors – murdering them, actually – but you get my drift: there are different ways to get started. It's your choice.

Your personality, your mental readiness, and the urgency of your need to change will drive how you go about this. There is no right or wrong way. There are no paleo police. What version of a paleo life you live is entirely up to you. Here are two ways to start on the paleo path.

DO A THIRTY-DAY CHALLENGE

This is a concept popularized by paleo folks all over. The concept is to dive into paleo cold-turkey for thirty days and experience the outcome.

If you do this, your food addictions and the health benefits of the lifestyle should be clearly exposed. Once the thirty days are done, the unwillingness to give up your newly-found health along with the confidence and lessons you learned will hopefully propel you forward so you don't revert back to your old habits.

You know how I mentioned personality, readiness and urgency earlier when considering your style of getting started? A thirty-day challenge like this is for those who are decisive and committed, and who are in a place where they know they have to change, and who refuse to accept a life that is sick and intolerable any longer. They want to see results quickly. It's a great way to determine if you have a health issue you suspect is diet related, and the support structure and determination to see it through. Anyone who completes a strict, thirty-day challenge deserves a lot of respect. It's tough. And for many, it is life-changing.

GO GRADUALLY

PALEO SECRET #1: THE SPEED YOU TRANSITION TO PALEO DEPENDS ON THE URGENCY OF YOUR NEED. DON'T LISTEN TO CONVENTIONAL WISDOM, EVEN PALEO WISDOM: INDIVIDUAL CIRCUMSTANCES DRIVE INDIVIDUAL SOLUTIONS.

While thousands of people have completed thirty-day challenges, it doesn't work for, or appeal to, everyone. There are whole swathes of people who balk at the idea. It is too radical and overwhelming. It feels just like another "diet." It can feel like moving into deprivation mode, and maybe after a lifetime of restricting calories, this can send you over the edge.

Others don't have a compelling reason to change their eating habits and lifestyle – they know they could (and perhaps should) do better, but nothing terrible is going to happen in the short term if they don't. And then there's the idea that this is a "rest-of-your-life-style" change, and easing out of a typical junk-food, wheat-and-sugar diet is more sustainable over the long term than an explosive burst out of the starting blocks.

If you are one of these people, it might pay you to go slower. Certainly, do not get the idea that going cold paleo turkey is the only way to get into the lifestyle. Don't use that as an excuse to throw your hands up in horror and continue to munch away on peanut butter and jelly sandwiches. There is another way.

Instead, you can overcome the inertia by dropping one thing. Maybe it's wheat or replacing vegetable oil for coconut oil when you're cooking. Or you can add one food item you typically haven't eaten much in the past, such as avocado or bacon. You can eat more eggs. Or try new vegetables. Keep at it. Keep learning and refining, becoming more and more paleo over time. You can always do a thirty-day challenge when you're ready for it. You can evolve into this lifestyle; just don't take as long as evolution itself, okay?

BASE THE SPEED OF YOUR TRANSITION ON THE URGENCY OF YOUR NEED

If your child has behavioral issues that are threatening to cause them to be expelled from school, you might be better served by taking a radical approach to changing your diet. If your arteries are clogged and a bypass (or worse) beckons, fast and drastic is the way to go. But if you want to lose fifteen pounds or avoid the afternoon slump, you can go slower. Choose the approach that works best for you and your need.

PURGE YOUR PANTRY IN ONE CLEAN SWEEP

If you do a thirty-day challenge, and even if you don't, you will need to clean up your pantry. There are likely to be things in there that are not paleo; am I right? Breakfast cereals; pasta; cans of beans; sugary snacks – many things like this will have to go. Grab a trash bag and fill it up. Take it to the food bank or just trash it.

ALTERNATIVELY, USE NON-PALEO FOOD UP AND DON'T REPLACE IT

If you're like me, and the idea of throwing away food you've paid good money for is horrific, or you have a family who'd rather throw *you* out than the non-paleo food, simply use it up but don't replace it. When you go shopping, buy fewer non-paleo foods (or none!) and more paleo fare. Over time, your shelves will get emptier and emptier, while on grocery shopping day, your fridge will be full to bursting. This is what you want.

ASSEMBLE A RECIPE FOLDER

Or buy a cookbook. The main thing is for you to have easy access to simple recipes that you can use as prompts to provide you with delicious meals, especially in the early days. I particularly like the idea of assembling your own folder, because the process of searching for recipes and compiling your own book acts as a reminder that this paleo thing is a serious endeavor. I have a folder full of empty plastic sleeves into which I slip recipes once I've tested them out on the family and got a "thumbs up."

WRITE A LIST OF ACCEPTABLE FOODS

You don't want to leave anything to chance, and investing time in your paleo tools will help you. Power up your text editor of choice and your favorite browser, and do your research. Make up your own list of paleo-friendly foods. Stick it on your fridge, then put those items on your shopping list.

SET ONE GOAL ONLY

You still have your daily life to manage that, if you're like most people, is already brimming to overflowing. We can't fight on too many fronts at once, so when you're deciding where to focus with paleo, choose only one goal at a time. Get that goal down and then set the next one. Diet has by far the most effect on your weight and health, but don't restrict your goal to just losing pounds.

FOCUS ON BUILDING SKILLS

In the beginning, spend time building your skills around eating and staying paleo. Your goal might be to paleo-ize your breakfasts, or to get through the holiday season without a paleo breakdown. Other examples are to become comfortable with saying "No, thank you" in every non-paleo situation, or to plan your meals each week. Remember skills are important because willpower is a finite resource that easily gets used up during the stresses of the day. Instead, get skilled at avoiding, dealing with, and managing the temptations that come your way by using strategies outlined here.

TAKE BABY STEPS

Long journeys are made up of many, many small steps. Break things down until you come to a bite-sized chunk you can manage. Have a goal to do ten pull-ups, but can't do a single one right now? Do as many or as much as you can. Or watch videos looking for good pull-up form. Or practice your grip. Keep doing this day after day, pushing yourself just a little further towards your goal each time.

SCHEDULE "DON'T-HAVE-TO DAYS"

These are like mini-vacations, and they allow you to rest. They don't have to last a whole day, or even half a day, but do make sure you take at least an hour. During this time, don't do anything you don't want to. You don't have to clean your teeth, clean up, shower, do your chores, workout, etc. unless you genuinely want to. No guilt. You just do what you like for the time you've allotted. These mini-breaks are to allow you to keep your willpower stores intact. Plan them so that life doesn't get in the way. Ask someone to take the kids if you have little ones, plan on eating out, and schedule time in your calendar if you have a hard time relaxing. Whenever I do this, I tend to let everything pile up while I read or listen to podcasts and drink tea. About two o'clock in the afternoon, I find I spontaneously and willingly start completing the minor chores I let go earlier in the day. I'm happier, perfectly relaxed and chilled, and look forward to the next time I get to have another "don't-have-to day".

BUILD MEDITATION INTO YOUR DAY

Meditation builds gray matter in the pre-frontal cortex, and scientific evidence shows that meditation can increase attention span, sharpen focus, improve memory, and dull the perception of pain.[3] In other words, it can act to increase willpower, or restore

3   "Meditation as Medicine", Paturel, Amy M.S., M.P.H.

it if your tank is low. Try making it a daily practice.

DO SOME FORM OF EXERCISE EVERY DAY

Working out has many of the same benefits as meditation and can act as a willpower enhancer when you're low or reinforce that which you already have. But it doesn't have to be a major workout. Walking around the block, especially if you are new to paleo, is perfectly fine – don't overdo it in the beginning, or you'll deplete your willpower super-quick.

Getting Started Checklist

- ☑ Do a thirty-day challenge or

- ☑ Go gradually

- ☑ Base the speed of your transition on the urgency of your need

- ☑ Purge your pantry in one clean sweep or

- ☑ Use non-paleo food up and don't replace it

- ☑ Assemble a recipe holder

- ☑ Write a list of acceptable foods and pin it up

- ☑ Set one goal only

- ☑ Focus on building skills

- ☑ Take baby steps

- ☑ Schedule "don't-have-to days"

- ☑ Build meditation into your day

- ☑ Do some form of exercise every day

STAYING CONSISTENT

So, you've got started. Things are working out. You understand what you're supposed to be eating, you're feeling better, you're seeing results, and you've developed a new array of favorite recipes. You think you've cracked it, you can stay like this for the rest of your life, and Bob's your uncle – you're gonna look good naked, have boatloads of energy, an amazing sex life, and millions in the bank. How can you not? You have discovered the key to the secret of life – eat . . . real . . . food.

But then you see the doughnuts on the coffee room table; you were in a rush this morning and had no breakfast. Or your mom bakes your favorite cake for your birthday, the size of which is almost as big as her eyes as she beseeches you to eat the token of her deepest love. Or you get treated to a special meal in a fancy restaurant, and the thought wafts across your mind that you'd be insane to turn down this gastronomic opportunity – it's a once in a ~~month's~~ lifetime's chance; you owe it to yourself to enjoy it in full, dammit!

> TAKE CARE OF YOUR BODY. IT'S THE ONLY PLACE YOU HAVE TO LIVE.
>
> ~ JIM ROHN

Our paleo path has twists and turns, and bumps and holes. It is the nature of the thing. We will trip up, fall over, and get lost. But we can make our path smoother. Here's how to stick at it once the euphoria has worn off.

CARRY OUT THREE GOAL-SUPPORTING ACTIONS DAILY

Do you want to lose a certain number of pounds? Live without pain? Build muscle? Make sure you are clear on your goal – only one major goal at a time, remember – and refer to it daily. Put it up somewhere that's prominent or easy to pull out. Focus on it. Imagine living, having already achieved it. Write three actions you can do today to progress towards your goal and carry them out.

FIND A DAILY PRACTICE

It could be going for a walk after dinner, logging your foods, or journaling. Make it as active a process as you can: For example, commenting on a blog is more active than simply reading it. But most importantly, make it something you can do *every day*.

EDUCATE YOURSELF ABOUT PALEO CONTINUALLY

Read and reread paleo books and blogs. Learn as much as you can about how the body works from sources you trust. New information and books are coming out continually. Stay on top of the latest news.

DON'T EVANGELIZE

The negative feedback you will get will rock you, and not in a good way. Keep quiet and calmly go about your business. Respond to only genuine and respectful inquiries.

PRACTICE SAYING "NO" AND "THANK YOU."

Say these words and say them often. Many are not accomplished at saying "no", especially those of us who are people pleasers. Practice them; say them out loud as often as possible. Tim Ferriss, in his book *The 4-Hour Workweek*, suggests lowering resistance to a particular activity by simply doing it over and over. The more you do it, the lower your resistance to it becomes; the more practiced you become, the more successful you'll be. He's talking about cold-calling, asking someone on a date, and that kind of thing, but we're talking about saying one phrase consisting of three short words. So, start saying, "No, thank you" to lots of things: volunteer activities, nights out, parties you don't want to go to, and offers of hand-me-downs that frankly insult you. It can be anything you don't want, like, or need. Just practice those words, and soon you'll handle the discomfort you feel much better.

TALK TO YOURSELF LIKE YOU WOULD YOUR BEST FRIEND

If most of us talked to our friends the way we talk to ourselves, we'd soon find ourselves all alone! We set far higher expectations for ourselves than we do for others, and we often need to moderate them. Being paleo is one of many, many priorities that we're trying to address and balance. And from time to time, things go awry. So, when you find yourself steering off the paleo path and beating yourself up for that, sit yourself down and talk to yourself. Turn that negative voice around. You ate something you wish you hadn't? Be kind, be proactive, and work out why. Devise a strategy for next time. Then ask yourself, "Was that really the end of the world? What can I do better next time?" Do it gently and with patience. Remind yourself of what you're good at, your self-worth and then, like you would coaching a Little League baseball team, tell yourself to get out there again, facing the world with your head held high.

DO ANY MANNER OF SELF-DEVELOPMENT EXERCISES

Any kind of self-development exercise will, by its nature, put the focus on you. Invest time in developing yourself. Buy a book, go on a course, or hire a teacher. Use this time to learn a skill, go back to school, or see a therapist. And don't worry about what other people think. Make the best decisions that work for you. Operate in your own paleo bubble if necessary. If you make yourself bigger in your own life, those around you will have less influence on your thoughts and patterns.

LEARN FROM EVERY SITUATION

At first, living paleo requires you to learn new skills. So, if you are having trouble staying consistent, always reflect on the lessons of your paleo life. See what you can learn from every less-than-satisfactory situation rather than see it as a failure. If you ate non-paleo in an unplanned way, always relive the experience. And if it is difficult for you to do so, it is even more important that you do. There is a lot of learning to be done there. Consider what worked, what didn't, what were your triggers, what needs further work, and what ideas you have for designing your behavior for more success in the future?

IF YOU'RE LOST, ASK FOR DIRECTIONS

If you're stuck on something, get over the hump and do it. Ask where to find that coconut butter in the store. Not sure what CrossFit is? Ask someone who does it. Other things you can do: send a question directly to a paleo blogger; go on a forum; subscribe to a favorite website for updates. Learn, learn, learn. And don't be shy; most people are happy to help.

GET ENOUGH SLEEP

Unless you are an extreme body hacker, if you are operating on inadequate amounts of sleep, you're hosed. Getting enough sleep is fundamental to a paleo lifestyle, and if you're not getting enough rest, start there. Don't even think about losing weight or joining a CrossFit box. Work on this before you tackle anything else.

MAKE EXERCISE EASY

Throw a few exercise toys around your house – not literally, of course; that would be counter-productive. Put up a pull-up bar in your kitchen. Keep a kettle bell in your bedroom. Sprint along your street. Wear sports clothing whenever you can, so you are ready to flex a few muscles whenever the opportunity presents itself. Be alert to exercise opportunities wherever you are, and exploit them.

Staying Consistent Checklist

- ☑ **Carry out three goal-supporting actions daily**

- ☑ **Find a daily practice**

- ☑ **Educate yourself about paleo continually**

- ☑ **Don't evangelize**

- ☑ **Practice saying "No" and "Thank you"**

- ☑ **Talk to yourself like you would your best friend**

- ☑ **Do any manner of self-development exercises**

- ☑ **Learn from every situation**

- ☑ **If lost, ask for directions**

- ☑ **Get enough sleep**

- ☑ **Make exercise easy**

BEING SUCCESSFUL

You're now ready to power this paleo lifestyle. Really take it up another notch. You want to learn advanced skills to take you to the next level and reap the rewards promised you.

Know that there are no shortcuts. Instead, focus on the bigger picture, on what's important to you, on what will give you long-term health and happiness. The following ideas will bring the results of your focus home to roost.

HAVE A WARRIOR MINDSET

Anticipate and train for every eventuality; be on the alert for danger every time you are faced with a situation involving non-paleo food. Know that this might be pretty much all the time in the beginning.

> HEALTH IS THE THING THAT MAKES YOU FEEL THAT NOW IS THE BEST TIME OF THE YEAR.
>
> ~ FRANKLIN P. ADAMS

But over months, and with practice, as a highly trained paleo warrior, you can keep on alert status without it being first and foremost in your mind. Sensing paleo danger will become second nature, and after a while, you will begin to intuit the danger and quickly go into "distract and refocus" mode and, later, complete indifference. Develop a list of behaviors and strategies for handling every non-paleo eventuality – dessert time at a dinner party; a friend's birthday; your partner's favorite cookies on the pantry shelf. Review this list often. Survey your territory frequently, and practice your defensive moves at every opportunity.

OBSERVE YOUR TRIGGERS AND ELIMINATE THEM

Every time you eat non-paleo in a way you don't feel in control of, analyze the situation. What set you off? What happened just prior to you eating? It may have been a tactical error – perhaps you stood next to the buffet table at a party. Or it might have been emotional – your boss/spouse/child/in-laws were pushing your buttons, and you went for the tub of frosting at the back of your pantry to calm yourself. Break the situation down into its component parts, looking for pieces that you can change or eliminate. Come up with strategies you can add to the situation to avoid seeking out non-paleo food – stand on the opposite side of the room from the party food; go for a walk; lock yourself in the bathroom for a couple of minutes; breathe deeply; journal. Keep analyzing your paleo faileos and develop new strategies until your avoidant behavior becomes automatic.

KNOW YOURSELF WELL

Are you are an "abstainer" or a "moderator"? This is highly important and easy to identify. An abstainer can't eat a moderate amount of a particular food – it's an all-or-nothing position to be in. A moderator can eat a small portion and stop. A moderator can eat a couple of squares of chocolate and put the bar down, while an abstainer would feel tortured by this limit, often feeling worse than eating no chocolate at all. An abstainer, once started, resists hugely the idea of stopping until completely satisfied (usually a thousand calories later) but might have a limit where they can stop without trouble. It is probably a very small amount – for me, it's a bite, just one, no more – but if you know what it is, it gives you a degree of flexibility and a boundary to work within. If you know yourself in this way, you can plan your strategies for dealing with non-paleo food much more effectively.

BE PREPARED

You cannot wing it with paleo until you're so practiced that it's automatic, and even then it isn't a great idea. You need to think ahead, plan your meals, and shop with those meals in mind. Know what you are going to eat in the days ahead. Set a time every week to plan. Make up a list from your plan, and go shopping. At the end of each day, plan the following day and review the meal plan to see what's left of your week so you are mentally and practically prepared for the following days. Complete the items you need to – take out frozen meat for thawing, rub a joint in preparation for tomorrow morning's crockpot, etc.

PALEO SECRET #2: DON'T LET THE PERFECT BE THE ENEMY OF THE GOOD. REVERSING LIFELONG EATING HABITS IS OFTEN ABOUT HAVING CONFIDENCE IN YOUR ABILITY TO CONTROL YOUR EATING. BUILD THAT CONFIDENCE BY NOTICING YOUR PROGRESS. YOU ARE MUCH MORE LIKELY TO STAY THE PALEO COURSE BY FEELING PROUD OF YOURSELF THAN BEATING ON YOUR OWN BEHIND TO FORCE YOURSELF ALONG.

GET SUPPORT

Are you always the weird one? Paleo peeps often are, unless they are fortunate to live in an environment of like-minded people. A relatively "new" lifestyle such as paleo attracts early adopters at this point in its development – those who are non-conformist and risk-takers, even if they look pretty conventional. So, pat yourself on the back for being so rad! The downside is it can get lonely, and there is little support from those around you. Even the greatest mavericks had moments of doubts and weakness, I'm sure, so to prevent this happening and to get help when it does, have a paleo world that you can dip into as you go about your day. Frequent paleo forums, attend (and host) paleo meet-ups, and dip into your purse or wallet for a few dollars to attend a seminar if there's one in your area. Believe me, it's worth it for the feeling of solidarity alone. Comment regularly, daily if possible, on your favorite blogs and their Facebook pages. Ask questions and develop relationships with those bloggers who reach out.

CREATE A PALEO OASIS

This is bit like the idea of having a shed or a cave to retreat to. Because we are faced with non-paleo threats at every turn, and especially if we have non-paleo food in our home, make sure you carve out a place to go relax that has no temptations. For me, it's my sauna. It might be your bedroom or perhaps your car. Or you can simply lie on the floor and close your eyes. Whatever it is, make it paleo-friendly. Definitely don't take non-paleo food along with you.

EXPERIMENT, EXPERIMENT, EXPERIMENT

Paleo guidelines are a baseline. From there, work out your own personal paleo prescription if you are not at your goal. Try different paleo combinations: drop nuts; go dairy-free; go fruit-free; research elimination diets. If you notice a reaction to a particular item, even if it falls within paleo guidelines, drop it and see for yourself how you get on. Make sure you note down symptoms beforehand and afterwards. Keep tweaking and testing; it may take months, but keep your eye on the prize in mind – great health – and keep on, keepin' on.

BE A PRO

Whatever it is you focus on, be excellent at it. If you choose to have a paleo lifestyle, make a commitment and then resolve to be professional about it. You might have an amateur skill set in the beginning, but with effort and training, you can become an expert. Resolve to get better and better.

WRITE DOWN YOUR SUCCESSES

Every day, week, or month, write down your successes. Reflect on them. Consider how far you've come. What works better in your life now? What negative aspects of your life have disappeared? Remember to take a medium-term view. Are you doing better this month than last, or than six months ago? If you are, congratulate yourself. If you're not, work out what is tripping you up. Find your triggers. I find that bacon makes me crave sweets later in the day. Who knew? You won't find that in any paleo handbook. That's the detective work you can do for yourself.

BECOME PUBLICLY ACCOUNTABLE

State your intentions out loud and put a system in place for holding yourself to account. Start a blog. Log your foods. Find a paleo buddy. Join a group. Don't be one of those people who are all talk and no action. Follow through and have a system, preferably a daily practice, to keep you accountable. State out loud and in print what you're going to do. And keep updating your public.

CHART YOUR PROGRESS

Measure something, anything: inches; macronutrients; fitness performance; whatever makes sense in relation to your goal. Monitor your progress daily, weekly, and monthly.

BREAK DOWN YOUR LARGER GOALS INTO BABY STEPS

Write down each baby step and check them off as you achieve them. Stick your progress sheet where you can see it and review it regularly. Observe how you're achieving and completing your goals.

MAKE PALEO YOUR PASSION

THE HIGHER YOUR ENERGY LEVEL, THE MORE EFFICIENT YOUR BODY. THE MORE EFFICIENT YOUR BODY, THE BETTER YOU FEEL AND THE MORE YOU WILL USE YOUR TALENT TO PRODUCE OUTSTANDING RESULTS.

~ANTHONY ROBBINS

This is where you get to teach others about paleo. Remember in school how they made you teach someone else to solidify the learning? This is what you do here. You will learn so much if you use a talent of yours and find an outlet to teach paleo concepts. If you write, start blogging. If you make art, make something that will illustrate paleo ideas. If you're a programmer, build a paleo app. Get creative and come up with an idea. Use your skills to spread the paleo word and strengthen your own skills in the process.

PERSEVERE!

Perseverance is, ultimately, what will make you successful. That's the magic! One foot after the other. You fall down; you get up. You wander off; you get back on track. This is a change of lifestyle, not a temporary thing when you get to go back to how things were after a while. Going and being paleo is an evolutionary process, and it is likely you will change your eating, playing, exercising, and relating over months and quite possibly years. Keep at it, keep refining, keep questioning, and keep reinventing yourself.

"If we are facing in the right direction,
all we have to do is keep on walking."
— BUDDHIST PROVERB

Being Successful Checklist

- ☑ Have a warrior mindset
- ☑ Observe your triggers and eliminate them
- ☑ Know yourself well
- ☑ Be prepared
- ☑ Get support
- ☑ Create a paleo oasis
- ☑ Experiment, experiment, experiment
- ☑ Be a pro
- ☑ Write down your successes
- ☑ Become publicly accountable
- ☑ Chart your progress
- ☑ Break down your larger goals into baby steps
- ☑ Make paleo your passion
- ☑ Persevere!

DEVELOPING ROUTINES

Routines streamline our lives. They put those things that are essential to our smooth functioning on autopilot and build structure into our day. They force us to focus on our priorities – eat well, sleep, move, and relax – so that everything else can be built on top of these fundamentals. Here are twelve routines you should ideally have in place – make establishing these a priority.

MEAL PLANNING

Meal planning is essential. There are lots of tools around to help you, from the very basic to the extensive, but the most important thing is that you actually *do it*. Set aside some time each week to plan out your dinners. If you like to try new meals and need to buy ingredients for recipes, planning before you do your main grocery shopping for the week is a good idea. Each day, review your plan for the *next* day so that you are always ahead of the game and can get items prepared and out of the freezer if necessary. I have simple crib sheets for family meal planning and school lunches that I fill out on Sunday evening.

GROCERY SHOPPING

It might seem obvious, but having ingredients in the house is fundamental to your ability to flow paleo. So many of us don't plan ahead, find ourselves with little to eat, and shop several times a week because we have to, not because we want the freshest ingredients. Or we end up eating out or snacking on the non-paleo stuff in the house, defeating our good intentions. Make doing grocery shopping a priority and keep to a regular schedule. Have a set day each week when you do most of your shopping, for example. Visit the farmers' market on the same day each week. Order those items you buy online on the first of the month. Collect your CSA promptly. Figure out what works for you and do it at the same time each day/week/month. Scheduling it in your calendar is important too.

DINNER PREPARATION

Preparation is the key to eating paleo day in, day out. Paleolithic man couldn't do it on the hop very often, and neither can you. Get it all ready in the morning if you can – you're fresh and your blood sugar is likely stable, making it less probable that you'll eat as you cook. If you prepare earlier, then come dinnertime, when you are tired and hungry, all you have to do is turn it on and finish it off. Plan a batch-cooking day once a week or month where you devote yourself to making up meals to freeze. Daily dinner prep becomes very easy if you do that.

BEDTIME

Sleep, sleep, sleep. Nothing works well if you're short here. A routine is key to winding down before sleep. Set yourself a bedtime and plan backwards to get those key things you need to get done every day before bed into a routine and completed before your bedtime arrives. Your brain will become accustomed to the process and know what's coming. You'll relax, knowing that things are done and set for the morning.

MORNING WAKE-UP

Our early-morning wake-up routine ensures we get to the place where we make our contribution to the tribe on time – in other words, our work. These days, this will look different for everybody – for those of us who work at home, it can be a case of simply rolling out of bed, or it may involve all sorts of shenanigans such as putting on makeup or a long commute. Whatever your personal wake-up routine, make it the same every day – repetitive, ordinary, normalizing.

> IT IS NOT THE STRONGEST OF THE SPECIES THAT SURVIVES, NOR THE MOST INTELLIGENT THAT SURVIVES. IT IS THE ONE THAT IS THE MOST ADAPTABLE TO CHANGE.
>
> ~CHARLES DARWIN

EXERCISE

Set yourself up with an exercise routine. Hook yourself up with a group if you need accountability. Do something daily, even if it is only taking the dog for a walk or doing a specified number of push-ups. Don't discount light work; we all have to start somewhere: Work up to a goal by taking daily, incremental baby steps. Schedule it into your day and notice what time of day works best for you. If you find yourself skipping it, check in with yourself to see if it is planned at the right time of day.

HYDRATION

Keeping hydrated gets forgotten about in the hectic pace of modern life. We then find ourselves gasping later in the day having, instead, kept ourselves topped up via our preferred caffeine delivery mechanism. Fill up water bottles first thing in the morning and carry them with you wherever you go. Keep them in your car and swig at stop lights – it is amazing how well you can set yourself up for your day in this way.

RELAXATION

PALEO SECRET #3: BEING KIND IS PREFERABLE TO BEING PERFECT BUT SOMETIMES PERFECTION IS IMPORTANT. IF THE CONSEQUENCE OF BEING KIND IS DREADFUL, BE PERFECT. IF THE CONSEQUENCE OF BEING PERFECT IS INSIGNIFICANT, BE KIND.

Modern times are so fast-paced, busy, and filled with activity from dawn until way beyond dusk that we get seriously unbalanced if we're not careful. If you are prone to workaholism (and I'm counting all computer-based activities as "work" in this instance, because it is a drain on your mind and body), you may have to make unplugged relaxation a priority and fix a routine around it. It might be reading a chapter of a novel before bed, or getting absorbed in a hobby for an hour, or fifteen minutes of yoga, but it must be something that is nearly as good as sleep for you.

JOURNALING

Cognitive behavioral therapy relies on journaling to support all behavioral change, and it is an important component to introduce when you wish to change your eating habits. You can structure your journaling by asking yourself questions, or you can simply write a stream of consciousness – writing for a certain length of time or number of pages. You can review it later, or not, depending on your preference, but it is best done daily. If you find yourself resisting, it is likely you need to do more of it. Questions you can ask yourself: What are my goals? What's stopping me? What am I afraid of? Is this fear really true? What can I do to manage my fear? What happened? How was I feeling? What was the outcome, and how could I change that in the future?

GOAL MONITORING

You will manage what you measure, so whatever your goal is – smaller dress size; strength; more energy; days without sugar – it is important to monitor your progress. Log what you do. Use food logs, spreadsheets, and journals, and make it a habit. It will keep you focused and provide you with data you can mine when you need to make changes.

FINANCIAL MANAGEMENT

Paleolithic man probably didn't have to worry about this, but we do. Being responsible financial managers is essential to our successful modern-day life, so automate this process, either by paying bills electronically, or by reserving a regular slot in your weekly or monthly calendar to do it. Also, don't forget budgeting and monitoring your spending.

CLEANING

They probably didn't do much of this in Paleolithic times either, I'm guessing, but feeling pride in our surroundings is important and contributes to our ability to accomplish. Daily maintenance of our home is important to our well-being, and we should spend a few minutes or more tending to it. Have a daily routine for straightening up and cleaning. Establish some regular weekly tasks and bigger, more infrequent tasks on a monthly basis.

Developing Routines Checklist

- ☑ Meal Planning
- ☑ Grocery Shopping
- ☑ Dinner Preparation
- ☑ Bedtime
- ☑ Morning Wake-Up
- ☑ Exercise
- ☑ Hydration
- ☑ Relaxation
- ☑ Journaling
- ☑ Goal Monitoring
- ☑ Financial Management
- ☑ Cleaning

NOTES

(BECAUSE INVESTMENT IN YOUR
PALEO PROCESS IS NECESSARY.)

SECTION THREE:

LIVING PALEO EVERY DAY

ORGANIZING YOUR KITCHEN

Your kitchen is the hub of your paleo world. This is where you bring your food once you've ~~hunted it down~~ brought it home from the grocery store. The kitchen is where you store it, prepare it, and maybe even eat it. It's where you come when you want something to calm you, to provide you with solace and comfort. Occasionally, you might even want something that fills you up. The kitchen is the palace in your paleo kingdom.

PALEO SECRET #4: IF YOU GO TOO FAST, YOU TRIP UP. SLOW DOWN . . . RELAX . . . BREATHE.

How you organize your paleo palace is critical to your success. A surgeon prepares his operating room with ultimate precision so that he can focus on the main job at hand. He doesn't want anything to distract him. You must do likewise.

ORGANIZE YOUR FRIDGE BY FOOD TYPE

You want to do this so that you hone in on your paleo food every time you open the door. Train yourself to know where exactly your food is and to ignore the rest. Have shelves designated paleo or non-paleo. Or organize by dairy, meat, vegetables, and other. As you open the door, visualize the interior and what you're looking for. Laser in on the item you want and screen out the rest. Don't have the fridge crammed full of stuff, or this won't work; you don't want to be rootling around in there. Make sure your items are easily housed and have plenty of space around them. Keep bottles of non-paleo dressings and sauces in the door shelves – they don't catch the eye there.

HAVE YOUR PALEO COOKING TOOLS EASILY TO HAND

Ideally, keep your crockpot out on the countertop at all times. If you have to lift it in and out of a cupboard, you're likely to use it less often. Invest in your favorite cooking implements – a double-steamer, particular tongs, or something else you like – to encourage you to cook your own food, and make cooking low-maintenance and possibly even a pleasure. Organize your baking trays so they don't all clatter to the floor when you get one, usually the bottom one, out. For those tools you use regularly, make them easily accessible by storing them in wide-mouthed or purpose-built containers on the work surface. Or put them in a drawer that is easy to open and close, and where the tools lie on the flat bottom so you can search around easily for your implement. Group like items together – your herbs and spices, your tools, your food storage materials, etc.

STORE YOUR TOOLS IN THE AREA IN WHICH YOU USE THEM

This is so you aren't constantly walking back and forth. Keep the chopping boards *near* your main work surface, your pots *under* the stove top, coconut oil *next* to the stove top, oven gloves *next* to the oven, your mugs *near* your kettle, and so on. It seems obvious, but so many people don't do it. Notice when you're walking all around your kitchen to grab items and see if you can organize your storage options more efficiently.

KEEP INDEX CARDS ATOP YOUR FRIDGE

These are to write down your paleo "aha's" – those tactics you use to keep yourself on the paleo path. While you can be afflicted by these momentary insights anywhere, your kitchen is the place where they strike the most. Be alert to them, note them down in this book or write up your own paleo advice handbook. Refer to it often; you can even stand it on your cookbook holder when you're not otherwise using it. Or tap your techniques and tips into your phone. Handwriting, though, has an indelible quality to it. Investing in your paleo process like this will support you in making this a lifestyle rather than a "diet."

USE YOUR KITCHEN SURFACES WISELY

Your kitchen is full of flat surfaces, right? Your fridge and other doors are prime paleo real estate. Stick up motivating messages, photos, acceptable food lists, meal plans, and recipes all around, but especially on your fridge door. Use fridge magnets, sticky notes, and poster putty to stick up your messages. Make sure you change them frequently, because after a while your brain will screen them out, and they'll no longer be effective. I laminate motivational quotes and post them up on my cupboard fronts. When I take them down I use them as bookmarks.

BUY PLENTY OF MEAT AND FREEZE IT

Always have meat on hand and pull it out to thaw the day before you plan to use it. Consider buying an extra freezer if you have to. I've never heard of anyone regretting doing that. The payoff over years makes getting one economical, not to mention the convenience, especially if you pick one up relatively cheaply. Buy meat on sale and in bulk, including part shares of beef, pork, etc., for the cheapest price.

EMPTY YOUR PANTRY SHELVES

If you are paleo, most of your food will be stored in the fridge or freezer. A few tins, and some spices, oils, and nut flours are all that are likely to be on the shelves. All the sugar, rice, pasta, breakfast cereals, packages, etc. will be gone. My cupboards are almost bare! Be proud of all the new-found space and empty shelving. If not, perhaps you need to take a look and have a purge. Depending on your style, you may prefer to throw it all away at once or go slower by eating it up and not replacing it.

HAVE A PALEO COOKBOOK OUT IN CLEAR VIEW

Visual cues bring to mind knowledge that can get obscured by the urgency to meet other demands – the need for comfort, to quell hunger, to satisfy a sugar craving, etc. Get a bookstand and use it to hold your "go-to" paleo cookbook. It will act as a visual prompt and cue you to keep on track, as well as give you ideas in a pinch. Using cues like this reinforces the notion that paleo is a lifestyle. They give you reminders, nudges, and inspiration for when you're feeling shaky about the whole thing. Make your home, and especially your kitchen, a paleo oasis as much as you can.

PUT LIKE-WITH-LIKE

Store herbs and spices together, preferably in a drawer or on a shelf close to your main work surface. Paleo recipes often use a lot of herbs and spices that can take up space, and you want to avoid overly cluttering the countertop. Place frequently used items such as salt, coconut oil, and pepper next to the stove top. Group your canned goods, flours, and baking supplies together in the pantry or cupboard. Put your spares in the pantry or on a shelf along with your dry cooking ingredients.

STICK RECIPES ON YOUR DRY MIX CONTAINERS

If you use the same dry ingredients in a recipe you make frequently, mix them in batches so you don't have to do it each time you cook. Stick the recipe on the side of the container so you can easily grab the rest of the ingredients and make the remainder of the recipe up prior to cooking. This works especially well for early morning paleo pancakes when you're trying to save time and not at your most alert, but it also works for cake mix, and even flour mix for dipping fish or meat before cooking.

Organizing Your Kitchen Checklist

- ☑ **Organize your fridge by food type**

- ☑ **Have your paleo cooking tools easily to hand**

- ☑ **Store your tools in the area in which you use them**

- ☑ **Keep index cards atop your fridge**

- ☑ **Use your kitchen surfaces wisely**

- ☑ **Buy plenty of meat and freeze it**

- ☑ **Empty your pantry shelves**

- ☑ **Have a paleo cookbook out in clear view**

- ☑ **Put like-with-like**

- ☑ **Stick recipes on your dry mix containers**

GETTING ENOUGH SLEEP

I thought about putting this segment at the front of the book, because without adequate sleep, just about everything else in paleo is twice as hard, and sometimes nigh on impossible. Not getting enough sleep doesn't just create a lack of energy, it also leads to weight gain, stress, and mood swings – the list goes on and on.

Getting enough sleep is paramount. If you don't, everything is tainted – slightly or a lot. It's the fundamental brick upon which the rest of our quality of life is based, so even if you do nothing else mentioned in this book, work on this.

SET A BEDTIME

We think this is for kids, but we need to set out our own line in the sand even as adults, or we can go on and on and on filling up our time with busyness. Set yourself a bedtime and plan your evening back from that. You can even use an alarm to alert you to the time to go do your routine. Make bedtime a priority.

MOTIVATE YOURSELF BY THINKING AHEAD

You know how you feel when you wake up with the jolt of an alarm? You can't believe it, can you? You're groggy, bad-tempered, and hung-over with lack of sleep, a feeling that doesn't go away until lunchtime. Then think how you feel when you wake up naturally, maybe early in the morning before anyone else is up. You're refreshed, striding purposefully towards your day, accomplishing things before the rest of the world even starts moving. Think of this the night before and resolve to take action to make it happen.

CREATE A NIGHTLY BEDTIME ROUTINE

We have routines in the morning, so why not in the evening? Each step of this wind-down routine prepares us mentally for sleep. You can make it a short or long process, but the most important thing is to keep it the same each night so that your brain knows what's coming: tidy up; set breakfast; clean teeth; jammies; read; lights out; good night.

PREPARE FOR BED WAY BEFORE BEDTIME

We often stay up because we're too tired to go to bed! Sounds silly when I say it, but it's true. Get in your pajamas, brush your teeth, and do your tidying up routine if you do one, and do this at least an hour before you need to. *Then* you can relax, knowing that when the time comes, you just have to roll into bed.

KNOW YOUR CAFFEINE LIMIT

Don't drink caffeine for several hours before bedtime. Allow your body to clear it out. And that also includes chocolate. I don't drink tea after four o'clock for this reason. Some people can drink caffeine *ad nauseum* and have it not affect their sleep, but that's not a healthy thing.

MAKE YOUR BEDROOM A PLACE FOR SLEEPING

Make it a calm haven from the rest of your life. You want to be able to sit in bed and survey a room that is pleasant and relaxing. No mess, cables, or papers strewn around. If you do have your office in your bedroom, screen it off.

> HUNGER IS THE BEST SAUCE IN THE WORLD.
>
> ~ CERVANTES

BLACKOUT THE ROOM

Maternity nurses and parents swear by this trick. This is the best way to get the body producing melatonin, the hormone that prepares you for sleep. Ideally, there should be not a crack of light peeping through your drapes or blinds, but a less-than-perfect situation will still be more effective than street and house lights blazing through your windows and doors. If you're really psyched to go all out, you can put up blackout blinds.

TURN OFF THE BLUE LIGHT

Blue light will interfere with you dropping off to sleep. Turn off the lights and TV an hour before bedtime. Read by torchlight or use an electronic reader that isn't back-lit. Laptops, tablets, and smartphones emit blue light, so avoid using those, too. The further away from your face the source of light is, the less effect it will have on you. Watching TV in an otherwise dark room won't have as much effect as a back-lit e-reader, but be judicious.

GET UP AT THE SAME TIME EACH DAY

If you need to sleep in, you aren't sleeping enough. And if you sleep in, you're pushing your body clock out so that it will be harder for you to get to sleep at bedtime. So, get up at the same time each day, every day. It might be difficult at first if you aren't going to sleep early enough, but keep at it until your body adjusts.

FOR DAYLIGHT SAVING, ADJUST YOUR BEDTIME BY FIFTEEN MINUTES FOR FOUR NIGHTS

It will help with the discombobulation and allow your body to adjust slowly to the time change. This is something I did with twin babies, and it works just as well for adults. You can also use this tip to adjust to an earlier bedtime if you are a nightowl.

EXERCISE (OR NOT)

Some people swear they can't sleep if they exercise before bedtime. Others say it helps enormously. Work out which type of person you are. If exercising just before bedtime works for you, do something that makes your legs heavy – squats or leg lifts – and gets you breathing deeply. For me, that works like a dream and sends me *to* my dreams.

Getting Enough Sleep Checklist

- ☑ **Set a bedtime**
- ☑ **Motivate yourself by thinking ahead**
- ☑ **Create a nightly bedtime routine**
- ☑ **Prepare for bed way before bedtime**
- ☑ **Know your caffeine limit**
- ☑ **Make your bedroom a place for sleeping**
- ☑ **Blackout the room**
- ☑ **Turn off the blue light**
- ☑ **Get up at the same time each day**
- ☑ **For daylight saving, adjust your bedtime by fifteen minutes for four nights**
- ☑ **Exercise (or not)**

SHOPPING PALEO

Shopping is the modern equivalent of the foraging that Paleolithic man and woman undertook every day. But while Paleolithic man had dangers to face hauling home his food, in contrast, but potentially perhaps just as deadly, we have lots of distractions and complexities to deal with. Special deals on cupcakes can waylay us, while items such as fish that look like fish, are labeled as fish, but aren't necessarily fish at all can confuse us. We have to have our wits about us.

SHOP THE PERIMETER

The healthiest foods in supermarkets lie around the perimeter of the store. The unhealthiest, and most profitable, occupy the center. This means that your grocery store shopping strategy should be to religiously steer your cart along the edges of the store. Produce, fish and meat counters, and a little in the refrigeration section. That's it. Done. Fewer options means things are accomplished much quicker and with no equivocation. There is rarely a need to go up and down the inner aisles, except for perhaps the occasional specific foray to get staples. Boom, boom, boom! Your weekly shop is over.

STOCK UP ON DRY GOODS AND MEAT MONTHLY

If you get really organized, you can have weekly lists for fresh produce, and monthly lists for staples and food you can freeze, such as meat. Once a month (I do mine on the first Sunday of every month), add your monthly list to your weekly list and do a slightly larger grocery shop, buying items like flours, paper goods and cans of coconut milk. It is surprising how time-efficient this system is.

MAKE A LIST AND KEEP TO IT

If you shop the perimeter, you basically bounce from food department to food department very quickly, buying mostly the same things over and over. But if you are new to paleo, on a budget, buying for new recipes, or just tempted to stray into the middle sections, make a list. Build your shopping list up from your meal plan and make sure you refer to any new recipes for ingredients. That way, you have everything you need when it comes time to cook.

IGNORE SALE ITEMS AND LOSS LEADERS

They are rarely paleo. Make an exception if they are. I stock up on meat on sale. But otherwise, just breeze through with your eye on the prize, a shopping cart full of items on your list.

ENTER THE STORE THROUGH THE PRODUCE SECTION

If you put produce items in your cart first, it starts your shop off right. It builds confidence and a feeling of empowerment, especially while you are learning. And you are more likely to keep going the healthy route and not get drawn in by tempting displays or offers. If you have no other choice but to go through the bakery section, be aware that the piles of cookies and cakes placed before you are there for a reason – you are being manipulated into buying them. Be smarter than the marketing guys – outwit them. Keep your eyes focused on the back wall and walk straight through the bakery without stopping.

SHOP FARMERS' MARKETS

Support your local farms, get access to the finest and freshest produce in your area, get to know the source of your produce, and buy in-season fruit and vegetables, not those that have been hot-housed or transported across continents. These are all great reasons to shop your local farmers' market. They're fun, too. Take the kids. My kids enjoy ours more than I do!

SHOP THE MEAT STACK

Ideally, buy grass-fed, grass-finished beef, and other meats that have been raised by ranchers who provide superior care of their land and their livestock. If that isn't possible, buy the cleanest, best meat that's available and that you can afford, even if it's grain-finished. And if that's not possible? Just buy meat – whatever you can get, and eat it, obviously.

BUY AT LEAST SEVEN DIFFERENT VEGETABLES

One for every day of the week. Mix it up and try new ones. Find recipes for side dishes to make veggies more interesting. Really look at every vegetable in your local grocery store or farmers' market – it's so easy to skip ones you're not familiar with. Pick a new one every week, and have a go at cooking it. Even if you don't do this, make sure you have plenty of variety in your produce – different colors, types, tastes and textures.

DON'T GO TO THE STORE HUNGRY

Or, worse, with hungry kids. Simple. End of. Period. The end.

BE A SMART SHOPPER AND CONSIDER THE TRADE-OFFS

In general, buy the highest-quality food you can afford, but weigh the benefits. If it takes you time and gas to get to a farmers' market, compare the prices and the relative quality of your local supermarket produce, and weigh up the pros and cons. Another thing to do is to look online – you might be able to buy smarter without even leaving your home. Invest time up front in becoming a conscious and savvy consumer. It's worth it.

GIVE HIGH-QUALITY PRODUCE A HIGH PRIORITY

We can pay more for our food to stay healthy, or more for our healthcare when things go wrong. It makes sense to bet your money on your family's health and pay a little bit more for your food. You can minimize the financial damage by being prudent and budget-conscious, but even then, you may find that you're shopping bill is a little higher.

SO, HOW DO YOU JUSTIFY THIS TO YOURSELF OR YOUR SPOUSE?

You reframe the situation. Think about the health benefits you are getting, the savings in medications costs, doctors visit copays, and out-of-pocket expenses.

Consider:

- the lessons and healthy foundation you are providing your children, and even your grandchildren
- the additional income you can earn as a result of being on top of your game
- the life satisfaction
- the therapist sessions you're not paying for
- the life and financial costs of depression and behavioral issues you're not experiencing.

It's an easy decision when you think about it.

Shopping Paleo Checklist

- ☑ Shop the perimeter

- ☑ Stock up on dry goods and meat monthly

- ☑ Make a list and keep to it

- ☑ Ignore sale items and loss leaders

- ☑ Enter the store through the produce section

- ☑ Shop farmers' markets

- ☑ Shop the meat stack

- ☑ Buy at least seven different vegetables

- ☑ Don't go to the store hungry

- ☑ Be a smart shopper and consider the trade-offs

- ☑ Give high-quality produce a high priority

EATING OUT

To have complete control over what you put into your body, the best thing is just not to eat out. Even items on the menu that seem paleo-innocuous are probably cooked in vegetable oil, not grass-fed, drenched in a sauce, or contain gluten in some shape or fashion. And then there's the dangers of the bread basket, the dessert menu, and the alcohol to deal with. There's no doubt about it, when you eat in a restaurant, you have to give up some control over what you put into your body. You have to take a risk.

But eating at home all the time is unrealistic, impractical, and just not fun. So, what do we do to minimize the risk and avoid turning a restaurant meal from a pleasant social occasion into a paleo catastrophe you'll be paying for way after the bill has been settled?

SURVEY THE MENU BEFORE YOU GO

Go online and make your choices ahead of time. Skim the menu first, skipping entirely the sections headed sandwiches, pasta, etc. Then go deeper. Go over and over the menu, if necessary, eliminating dishes and considering possible substitutions for non-paleo ingredients and items. Have your requests prepared before you even arrive at the restaurant. And generally, I would recommend avoiding restaurants whose menus take twenty minutes to read – way too much distraction leading to potential overstimulation and poor choices.

ASK FOR SUBSTITUTIONS

When you get to the restaurant, ask for what you want, not the combinations they have put together – what *you* want. You are the paying customer. Just about every restaurant accommodates with substitutions, and if you find yourself in one that does not, vote with your feet and go elsewhere. Use this power and flexibility to ask for a plain salad instead of pasta, or spinach instead of fries, that kind of thing.

PALEO SECRET #5: YOU MANAGE WHAT YOU MEASURE. IF WE MEASURE, WE'RE NOTICING. WE'RE ANALYZING, AND WE'RE THINKING. WE'RE SLOWING DOWN AND ACTING LESS ON IMPULSE. WE'RE BECOMING CONSCIOUS OF OUR ACTIONS AND THEIR CONSEQUENCES. WE'RE MINDFUL. THESE THINGS MATTER. YOU MATTER. MEASURE, MANAGE, MATTER.

GET TO KNOW YOUR RESTAURANT

Surprise is the enemy of the paleo warrior, so avoid being distracted by a new and potentially vast menu; go to a restaurant you know and love. Frequent a few and become familiar with their offerings. As a regular patron, they might even start making dishes especially for you.

ASK FOR CUSTOMIZED MENU COMBINATIONS

This is a slightly bigger ask than substitutions, but for a restaurant interested in keeping their customers happy, it only demands an open mind and some flexibility. Make up your own meal by mixing and matching items from different dishes on the menu and see if your restaurant will accommodate you. For example, if they are offering eggs in one breakfast dish, and chicken and spinach in another, ask if they will give you a chicken scramble. They won't always do this, and if so, you needn't go back, but often they will, and you'll get a great meal.

REFUSE THE BREAD BASKET

Nothing undermines a paleo mindset like the ubiquitous bread basket. Grown women have been known to resist throughout a two-course meal only to cave in while waiting for their dinner partners to finish (that would be me). So, just keep it right away – wave it away, or put it well out of reach. Ask for your fellow diners' support in this.

HOLD THE BAGELS, TOAST AND HASH BROWNS

Ask for all the non-paleo items to be left off the plate. Don't waste your energy looking at them and having to resist them. Just don't have them arrive at your table.

MAKE A MEAL UP FROM A VARIETY OF SIDE DISHES

When you open up your menu, head straight for the side menu, especially if you want a smaller, less complicated meal. Make up a meal that works for you from the side dishes you find. It may be more pricey, but ultimately, it is worth it.

PICK A PLACE WITH SALADS

Even salads these days are non-paleo with their heavy dressings, candied walnuts, and strong cheeses, etc. But salads still offer a fairly safe bet for a paleo peep, especially if you go to a place with plenty of choice. Ask for your own combination of salad ingredients and *always* ask for your dressing on the side.

EXPERIMENT VISITING GRILLS, ROTISSERIES, AND ETHNIC RESTAURANTS

These types of restaurants may be more paleo-friendly, so try them out. Barbecued food is obvious, but did you know that Brazilian food can be really quite paleo? Greek, Japanese, and Peruvian cuisines also have some great paleo foods if you choose wisely, so try ethnic restaurants – you might be pleasantly surprised. (Conversely, it is my opinion that nothing good from a paleo perspective ever came out of an Italian restaurant, so be warned.)

CONVERT YOUR FRIENDS

There is no reason ever to eat off-paleo, or sound like you never got over your fussy-eater stage as a toddler, if you eat at home. Invite friends over for a meal instead of eating out – even if they're not paleo. Introduce them to all the wonderful paleo dishes on offer. You never know, they might become converts.

Eating Out Checklist

- ☑ Survey the menu before you go

- ☑ Ask for substitutions

- ☑ Get to know your restaurant

- ☑ Ask for customized menu combinations

- ☑ Refuse the bread basket

- ☑ Hold the bagels, toast and hash browns

- ☑ Make a meal up from a variety of side dishes

- ☑ Pick a place with salads

- ☑ Experiment visiting grills, rotisseries, and ethnic restaurants

- ☑ Convert your friends

HACKING BAG LUNCHES

Making up a bag lunch every day has got to be one of the most tedious chores that ever existed. It makes sense, both from a paleo perspective and a financial one – but yeah . . . ugh! I have found that systematizing the process makes for a better lunch, removes the daily frustration of having to come up with ideas, and lessens the likelihood that you'll abandon your good intentions and skip off to the sandwich shop. Consider these ideas to make it easier, and even fun!

TAKE A MODULAR APPROACH

Automate everything you can in order to keep it easy and happening. Make up a list of main dishes, consisting of proteins and a list of sides (mostly raw veggies). Stick it on your fridge. Pull one item from the "mains" column and at least two sides for every meal.

Mains	Sides	Desserts
• Leftovers • Spinach Meatballs • Chicken Drumsticks • Turkey Meatloaf • Sausages • Mini Frittatas • Hard-Boiled Eggs • Tuna or Salmon, Capers, and Home-made Mayo • Burger Patties	• Carrots • Tomato • Cucumber • Salad Greens • Peppers • Radish	• Fruit (especially berries) • Pumpkin Muffins • Banana Bread • Fruit and Nut Bars • Brownies

PLAN YOUR LUNCH WEEK

Just like you do for dinner (you do plan your dinners, don't you?), make a meal plan for your lunches. This takes out the "what-am-I-going-to-have-for-lunch-today?" questions and the wasted energy and worry as you stare and stare at the contents of your fridge, while your inspiration deserts you and your anxiety rises. The clock keeps ticking, and the moment of your departure gets closer and closer, but no ideas spring to mind. Instead of living through this scenario every morning, make up a planning sheet in your text editor of choice and fill it in weekly, or do what I do – scribble on a sticky note and attach it to your lunch food list.

CONSIDER NUTRITIONAL BALANCE OVER A WHOLE DAY

Occasionally, lunch will be light on veggies – we can get bored of raw vegetables, and warmed up veggies are just nasty, or you might have gotten low towards the end of the week. On those occasions, lunch might be a little protein-heavy or veggie-light, but that's okay; make up for it at breakfast or dinner. In our house, we have green smoothies in the morning; they are fantastic for you and make us feel sooooo paleo-worthy.

PREPARE YOUR LUNCHES IN THE MORNING

This is a highly personal preference, but spending ten minutes then is often easier, especially if you take a systematic approach. At the end of the day, making lunches for the next day can be a real pain, particularly if you're tired or tend to eat while you're prepping food. Another reason to do it first thing is that you really want the food to be as fresh as possible.

USE LEFTOVERS

Leftovers should be one of your lunch staples. They cut down on effort and thinking by a great amount. You'll need a thermos to keep them warm, so invest in one of those. Cooking a delicious paleo meal and making enough for dinner and lunch the next day with virtually no additional work is a win-win-win. Have leftovers at least three times a week.

USE DISPOSABLE CUTLERY

THE BODY IS LIKE A PIANO, AND HAPPINESS IS LIKE MUSIC. IT IS NEEDFUL TO HAVE THE INSTRUMENT IN GOOD ORDER.

~HENRY WARD BEECHER

I suggest using disposable cutlery, especially if you're sending them with kids to school. Too many times we lose our cutlery and some places will consider metal knives and forks weapons, so take cutlery such that, if you do lose it, it's not the end of the world. Remind kids to bring it home so it can be washed and reused. You can make one box of plastic cutlery last years that way. That's pretty efficient.

GIVE GENEROUS PORTIONS OF EACH SELECTION

This is to cut down on the number of different items you have in your lunch, which makes for less stress and mess. Aim for three to four different items total, maybe less.

GET KIDS INVOLVED IN PREPARING LUNCHES

If you only have paleo food in the house, it's easy as the kids get older to have them more invested in their lunch preparation. Have them roam your fridge and shelves to select what they want or have them choose from the "menu." They'll eat more if they have more choice in the matter. Even if they are little, they can still make choices such as "Carrots or celery?" And as they get older, give them more and more responsibility. At age twelve, my kids get their own "sides," while I prepare the "main course."

HAVE A "WATER-ONLY" RULE

Make water your friend. Water can seem plain after drinking soda or other flavored drinks, so I suggest sticking to water only, especially for kids. After a while, you'll stop thinking of drinking anything else. Water bottles with sports tops are the easiest to drink from, and you'll drink more if it's easy to do so. Make it a practice to drink from them regularly and set yourself a water-drinking principle – drink at every stoplight, on the hour, or each time you take a work break, for example.

DESSERTS ONLY OCCASIONALLY, OR NOT AT ALL

Treat desserts as an occasional indulgence, even for kids. Don't pack them with any regularity. If you do take a dessert, make it something like a piece of fruit, a paleo muffin, or a couple of dates.

Hacking Bag Lunches Checklist

- ☑ Take a modular approach
- ☑ Plan your lunch week
- ☑ Consider nutritional balance over a whole day
- ☑ Prepare your lunches in the morning
- ☑ Use leftovers
- ☑ Use disposable cutlery
- ☑ Give generous portions of each selection
- ☑ Get kids involved in preparing lunches
- ☑ Have a "water-only" rule
- ☑ Desserts only occasionally, or not at all

STAYING ON BUDGET

While eating paleo isn't the cheapest way of eating out there (until you factor in healthcare, that is, and then it becomes dead cheap), there are many things you can do to limit your costs. I found that once I'd got clear about how I shopped, I spent no more in Whole Foods than I had when I'd gone to Safeway.

As with anything, it all depends on what you're willing to forsake and the choices you make. With a little bit of effort and some due diligence, you can make big inroads into your monthly food bills and keep it to a reasonable level.

HAVE A BUDGET AND MONITOR IT

Track what you spend on food for a couple of months – you might be surprised. Simply becoming aware in this way is helpful, but if you want to go to the next step, write everything down (or buy everything with a card and review your monthly bank statement) and put your expenses into a spreadsheet. Examine it every month and see where you can make savings.

CHALLENGE YOURSELF TO KEEP TO A CERTAIN FOOD EXPENDITURE EVERY MONTH

This is great to do with the kids and teaches them so much. In our family, we make guesses on what our food bill will come to based on what we lay out on the checkout conveyor belt. At first we'd be way off, but after a while we got pretty accurate. We keep track of how much we spend each week, and on the last week of the month, we make sure we only spend what we have left in our monthly budget. It is amazing how resourceful you become under pressure!

BUILD IN SOME CREATIVITY TO MAKE IT FUN

Look for new recipes with cheaper paleo foods, and subscribe to paleo blogs and sites that have this kind of advice. Try new recipes regularly to build up your collection of budget meals. If you make some recipes up of your own, put them in an eBook and sell them, making yourself some money in the process – with which you can buy some more paleo food! Alternatively, Robb Wolf has an eBook, *The Paleo Diet Budget Shopping Guide,* that has a lot of great advice. It will pay for itself in the first week.

BUY CHEAPER CUTS OF MEAT

Ground beef is your friend. Stewing steak can be delicious in a casserole, especially when combined with some "two-buck chuck" from Trader Joe's. And use a crockpot. There's just no way round it, you've got to have one. You can make the most delicious meals with the cheaper cuts, even offal doesn't taste "offal."

VISIONS AND DREAMS ARE ACHIEVED THROUGH TAKING SMALL STEPS, DELAYING GRATIFICATION, AND USING STRATEGIC THINKING.
~UNKNOWN

BUY PALEO ITEMS ON SALE

Be a smart shopper and look for food on sale, especially meat. Buy as much as you can afford at these times and store it. Don't ignore places like Whole Foods, even if you think it is "whole pay-check." They have some great one-day deals, so keep an eye out, but don't get distracted by non-paleo bargains!

COWPOOL

Great meat for a great price. You can buy all kinds of cuts of grass-fed and finished beef for less than the price of ground meat in the store. If you can't afford the up-front cost of a part share, ask the rancher if they sell cuts in smaller quantities. Often they will, and while it will be more expensive per pound than if you bought a larger amount, it will still be cheaper than store-bought meat. Check out the Eat Wild website in the Resources section to find a rancher near you.

DO IT YOURSELF

Where you can, prepare and grow your own food; it's always cheaper and better quality. Paleo meals and baked goods you already make, I'm sure, but have you tried making sauerkraut, kombucha, or your own chicken stock? Or rendering lard or tallow from your cowpool meat? Try it. You'll find out how quick, easy, and delicious it is, and you'll never think of buying it again. I wouldn't dream of buying stock in a carton or can now – it's so easy to make, and satisfies my thrifty nature. Compost. Grow vegetables. Raise chickens. Once you start changing your lifestyle to paleo, there is always more you can do, and more savings you can make.

JOIN A CSA

Community Supported Agriculture (CSA) has become a popular way for consumers to buy local, seasonal food directly from a farmer. The food is often cheaper, fresher, and of higher quality than store-bought produce, but be careful to make sure you are buying a box that meets your needs. Don't get too large a box with so much produce that you can't keep up with it and ultimately end up wasting it, and make sure you aren't getting so much produce that you can't or won't eat it. Share your box with a friend if you need to. Check out the Local Harvest website in the Resources section to find a CSA near you.

FAST

Seriously. Skip a few meals. It adds up. And it will support your health. Make intermittent fasting part of your schedule.

Check out the section on I.F. in *The Primal Blueprint* or on Marks Daily Apple.

BUY IN QUANTITY TO GET SAVINGS

If you have paleo friends, you can go in together. You can buy coconut oil in five gallon pails from Tropical Traditions, for instance. And you can sign up for Subscribe and Save on Amazon.com, and get discounted prices and free shipping.

AVOID PALEO BAKED GOODS

Baked goods cost a lot to prepare relative to other foods in your paleo shebang, and there are better ways to spend your money from a nutritional perspective. Put your money into protein and produce; they will give you more nutritional bang for your buck.

CUT DOWN ON OTHER EXPENSES

It doesn't cost anything to walk or exercise at home. It's cheaper to camp than cruise, and to have friends over than eat out. Look at how you spend your time and money. Analyze your expenses spreadsheet and switch out costly activities for cheaper ones. Save your money for that which you put in your bodies.

SORT OUT YOUR PRIORITIES AND VALUES

There is always a price to be paid. Good quality food costs money. Poor quality food costs good health. Buying in bulk costs less in the long run, but more up-front. Decide what you can do, and what you're willing to pay. In other words, establish your priorities and decide on your trade-offs. If you do that, budgeting decisions come easy.

REMEMBER PALEO-*ISH* IS STILL WAY BETTER THAN A CONVENTIONAL DIET

Don't let perfection be the enemy of the good. Don't let your inability to eat 100 percent paleo all the time cause you to throw up your hands and give up. You may not be able to be hard-core paleo – eating grass-fed and finished, raw and organic – but it's still much better than the alternative. Do what you can with what you have. And keep striving.

Staying on Budget Checklist

- ☑ Have a budget and monitor it
- ☑ Challenge yourself to keep to a certain food expenditure every month
- ☑ Build in some creativity to make it fun
- ☑ Buy cheaper cuts of meat
- ☑ Buy paleo items on sale
- ☑ Cowpool
- ☑ Do it yourself
- ☑ Join a CSA
- ☑ Fast
- ☑ Buy in quantity to get savings
- ☑ Avoid paleo baked goods
- ☑ Cut down on other expenses
- ☑ Sort out your priorities and values
- ☑ Remember paleo-ish is still way better than a conventional diet

NOTES

(BECAUSE YOU DON'T HAVE TO DO
WHAT OTHER PEOPLE TELL YOU.)

SECTION FOUR:

LIVING PALEO –
UNUSUAL SITUATIONS

GOING ON VACATION

Being away from our kitchens, our routines, and our local grocery stores can throw even the most hard-core paleo-istas for a loop. Add to that mix the fact that we might be in the middle of nowhere, eating only what we've brought with us, or conversely, in the midst of a cornucopia of culinary delights, the majority of which are sadly but decidedly **not** paleo, and we have a complex situation. All our regular eating habits and resolutions can go out the cruise ship window.

Vacations offer a particular challenge, both in terms of eating paleo and resisting temptation. Away from home, it's easy for our eating habits to go on vacation along with the rest of us. But there are steps you can take to avoid experiencing a paleo vacation disaster. Consider these:

PLAN A *PALEO* VACATION!

Keeping paleo on vacation starts before you've even booked your trip. Think ahead and consider how you might add as many paleo elements into your vacation as possible – food and exercise – especially moving slowly and often, sleep, and play. For some, a decision will involve camping in the woods, cooking over a campfire, and spending days rollicking around in nature. Maybe you choose that kind of vacation over a cruise or a trip to Disneyland, but even on those twenty-first-century non-paleo idylls, you can still build paleo elements into your time away.

SCOUT YOUR ENVIRONMENT AS SOON AS YOU ARRIVE

PALEO SECRET #6: IF IN DOUBT, KEEP QUIET.
PLAY SAFE, TALK LESS, AND OBSERVE.

If you're traveling around on vacation, you're going to be doing a lot of reconnaissance, but it is necessary if you are to manage your eating. You need to look for the places that will provide you with good foods – supermarkets, farmers' markets, and an acceptable restaurant. And you need to look out for the threats – the pizza joints, the teashops, and the roadside food stalls – so you can anticipate them and work out your strategies. Keep your eyes open and be watchful.

THINK AHEAD AND STRATEGIZE

To manage the threats to your paleo principles, plan your strategies out. If you've done some reconnaissance and surveyed the lay of the land, you'll have identified the potential problems. Plan out how you will address those threats. Maybe you'll survey an area, deciding what and how much you'll consume. Maybe you'll plan your eating stops and check out a restaurant menu ahead of time. Or eat before you go. Or take your own food in. Just think ahead and make up a defensive plan.

COOK YOUR OWN FOOD

Whenever you eat out, you are taking a paleo risk. Non-paleo ingredients and cooking methods can make restaurant food highly questionable. The fact that you haven't invested in the preparation of your food and are possibly focusing on other aspects of the meal, such as socializing, makes it more likely that you will make poor choices. There is the visual temptation of the dessert menu and the lack of familiarity with new places to contend with, too. All in all, restaurant dining is fraught with danger for a paleo peep, and being on vacation compounds that danger. The more you can lower that risk, the better. The safest bet when choosing a paleo vacation is to plan one where you make your own food as much as possible. Even better, plan a vacation that allows you to cook like you would at home. Rent a suite, a cottage, a trailer, or a barbecue pit – anywhere where you can easily cook your own food.

PLAN YOUR MEALS LIKE YOU DO AT HOME

Take your routines away with you on vacation. Pack them in your bag with your swimsuit. Use a simple paper planner, plug in your meals *before you go*, and make shopping lists as necessary. Plan on making the same foods as you do at home and adapt as necessary while on your trip. If you are eating out some, and you probably are, batch-cook multiple portions of the same meals when you get there, and eat them spaced out in between restaurant meals for variety.

TREAT YOUR COOKING TOOLS AS DISPOSABLE ITEMS

Cooking while on vacation is much easier, and you are more likely to do it if you have your favorite cooking tools. If you are going on a road trip, take them with you. If you are flying, buy them when you get there and leave them behind when you go home. Don't worry about the cost – doing this is a lot cheaper than eating out. On my last trip, I bought a crock pot, steamer, and tongs. I get frustrated, and therefore more likely to throw in the towel, without them. Cooking paleo on vacation becomes a lot more enjoyable with my favorite tools.

EXERCISE

Don't worry about your usual workout (unless you really want to), but look for ways to build exercise into your day. Identify vacation activities that require you to be active, not passive. You can always build walking with your loved ones into your day wherever you are.

BE A SMART AIR TRAVELER

A MAN TOO BUSY TO TAKE CARE OF HIS HEALTH IS LIKE A MECHANIC TOO BUSY TO TAKE CARE OF HIS TOOLS.

~SPANISH PROVERB

Eat a big paleo meal before you go with a good amount of fat. Prepare your own food for the flight, make more than you think you'll need (it's boring just sitting there), and just toss it if you have any left on your arrival. Ignore the airplane food. Take a large, empty water bottle on board and have the crew fill it up for you. Use the free eye shades or take some with you and get some sleep.

PACK PALEO-FRIENDLY SNACKS

As you are wandering ruins or climbing the stairs to Space Mountain for the fifth time that day; it is good to know that in your pocket you have food to stave off the hunger pangs. Nuts, jerky, or cut-up veggies will get you through to your next healthy meal, without having to resort to the immediacy of the carb-laden roadside food carts or a local fast-food option, if you are overcome with hunger. Of course, if you have a good paleo breakfast before you go, you should be good for hours and hours. And then there's always fasting . . .

REMEMBER THE "MEAT-AND-VEG" MANTRA

You can't go wrong if you stick to meat and veg. Don't over-complicate things, especially on vacation. When you shop or peruse a menu – the modern version of foraging – keep these three little words in mind in order to make good choices. If something doesn't fall within these parameters, move on. Repeat after me: "Meat and veg: meat and veg: meat and veg . . ."

ENJOY YOURSELF!

Have some fun. Don't hold yourself in check like a tightly wound coil. The paleo police aren't going to come and get you. Really. Decide if, when, where, and how much you will allow yourself off-plan. Consider the consequences of doing so and make your plans accordingly. I sometimes allow myself off-paleo for the last day of my vacation. Or I'll make a list of the things I must try, then I halve the list and savor one (but only one) of each item during my time away. This might be an especially good idea if it stops you going off the deep end (and I'm not talking about the hotel swimming pool).

Going on Vacation Checklist

- ☑ **Plan a paleo vacation!**
- ☑ **Scout your environment as soon as you arrive**
- ☑ **Think ahead and strategize**
- ☑ **Cook your own food**
- ☑ **Plan your meals like you do at home**
- ☑ **Treat your cooking tools as disposable items**
- ☑ **Exercise**
- ☑ **Be a smart air traveler**
- ☑ **Pack paleo-friendly snacks**
- ☑ **Remember the "meat and veg" mantra**
- ☑ **Enjoy yourself!**

GETTING THROUGH THE HOLIDAYS

U gh. This can potentially be a nightmare. The challenge starts at Halloween and, depending on your viewpoint, goes through December, possibly January (Super Bowl), and even February (Valentine's). Oh, I nearly forgot, there's Easter. And Mother's Day. And birthdays. And because "it's Friday." Any excuse. It goes on and on.

We exist in a perpetual holiday state, and we have to deal with the onslaught of all those celebratory foods that we as a culture have somehow come to associate with those days.

LIMIT THE HOLIDAYS YOU CELEBRATE

You can find a reason every week to celebrate if you want to. Instead, question how much you really have to celebrate each and every holiday that comes up. As an adult, I don't celebrate Halloween, the Super Bowl, Valentine's Day, Easter, or July 4th with any kind of special food. I eat what I normally eat. That still leaves me Thanksgiving, Christmas, my birthday (and those of my immediate family), Mother's Day, and vacations to celebrate with food, and that's more than enough.

Use holidays to look at your relationship with food and examine if it's really necessary to celebrate with a feast or if there's another way, or simply skip it entirely.

PLAN AHEAD AND DEFINE YOUR LIMITS

Ahead of time, decide what you're going to allow yourself. What will you eat and when? What will your strategies be for keeping on track? You must know the answers to these questions and have a plan of action in place. Anticipate and think how the upcoming celebration will play out – plan your meals and define your indulgences, if you plan to have any. Once you know if you are an abstainer, use all the strategies that are contained in this book and those you have worked out for yourself to keep you on the straight and narrow.

HAVE A RECOVERY PLAN IN PLACE

If you decide you are going to go on a vacation from paleo and eat whatever you want, run through the consequences of doing that and have a recovery plan. Make sure you know ahead of time what tomorrow and the next days might look like, and make a decision as to whether it is worth it and if it's sensible given what you have planned in the next few days. If you do decide to go ahead, plan now for how you will get back into paleo mode. Will you fast the next day? Snap right back into paleo? Sleep it off? It's the same as considering whether to drink alcohol – you think ahead and weigh the consequences. (See the section on Climbing Back on the Paleo Wagon for more ideas.)

UNDERSTAND YOUR REACTION TO ALCOHOL

Alcohol acts as an appetite enhancer, as well as causing us to be more impulsive. A planned alcohol indulgence can become a full-on binge for some people, both in terms of drink and food, so know your limits and act accordingly.

TAKE YOUR OWN FOOD

If you're attending a potluck, make sure there's something for you to eat. Maybe several things – a main dish and a dessert. It's incredibly satisfying to see non-paleo peeps scarf a paleo dish and a great way to introduce people to paleo without them even realizing!

BE THE HOST

Hosting means you define the food agenda. And it isn't difficult to make a paleo Thanksgiving, for example. Just hold the bread rolls and make sweet potato mash. After a second, no one will even notice the usual suspects are missing. Even if someone insists on bringing non-paleo food (I can just hear someone announcing "It's not Thanksgiving without the rolls!"), you can guarantee that by hosting the meal, it is far more paleo than it would have otherwise been. And when they eat the best paleo desserts, no one will bother that the usual pies are absent. Best of all, you get loads of food that *you* can enjoy!

RETHINK THE EMPHASIS ON FOOD AT HOLIDAY TIME

Our house used to be full of chocolate on Christmas. It was on the tree, in tins to eat in front of the TV, in the kids' stockings, and behind the doors of the advent calendar. And then we had many, many cakes, pies and other goodies that filled our days long before and for a short while after "the day." It was unconsciously excessive and totally ridiculous once my eyes had been opened. That has all gone, and in its place . . . nothing. We eat a paleo breakfast and eat out for dinner. The next day, we are back to eating our regular paleo diet. All this excess is just . . . excess. It doesn't enhance our experience beyond a certain point, and we don't miss it when it's gone. Consider what changes you can make so that food doesn't feature so much in your celebration.

KEEP MOVING

Earn your dinner. Develop an appetite. Go out in the morning and get active. Take the kids/dog/guests for a hike. Play an outdoors game. Snowshoe. Just wrap up warm and get outside. Be active. Then enjoy your dinner.

AVOID STORES THE DAY AFTER A HOLIDAY

You know, those days after Christmas, Valentine's Day, Easter, Halloween, etc., when the drug store is off-loading what's left. You can get chocolate *and* save money! That used to be my kind of bargain. We often keep buying and buying more food at holiday time. Cut-price candy, chocolate, and other goodies in particular will tempt us to buy more, more, more. This is especially so if our sugar levels are all over the place because we've been eating non-paleo in the preceding days. So, make sure if you go into the store, you don't go down the candy aisle. Visualize it before you get there and plan your route around the store so you don't go down where the candy is displayed. Even better, don't go in the store in the first place. Go somewhere else, such as a park.

FAST WHEN YOU CAN

Skipping a meal can make all the difference. You certainly won't starve. Pick a meal you can reasonably do without and go out for a hike instead.

STAY FAR AWAY FROM THE PARTY TABLE

Go in a different room, stand with your back to the table, put several people between you and the food, and concentrate on them. However you do it, keep well away from the feast and avoid the visual stimulation that will pull you in. And seriously consider staying away from parties entirely. If you don't particularly enjoy them and they tend to make you haunt the buffet like the Ghost of Christmas Past, be very selective about the ones you go to, or give them a pass entirely. Life is too short to do things you really don't want to do or that will make you feel bad for hours afterwards.

COMMUNICATE, DON'T CONSUME

Big events *always* involve food, there's just no getting around it. Family reunions, especially, are highly likely to contain a plethora of non-paleo food along with quite a few paleo skeptics, noticing and judging what you eat. Added to that, they're often an emotional minefield which, when combined with rare meet-ups and long memories, make for stress leading to a potential paleo disaster. Keep on the down-low with your eating, I say. Concentrate on socializing pleasantly and hold off on the eating for as long as possible. Just quietly eat what you can and don't make a big fuss. Don't focus on the grand food plate in front of you. Enjoy your companions, take the emphasis off the food, and walk away from those looking to pick a fight or being otherwise obnoxious. You don't need the aggravation.

Getting Through the Holidays Checklist

- ☑ Limit the holidays you celebrate
- ☑ Plan ahead and define your limits
- ☑ Have a recovery plan in place
- ☑ Understand your reaction to alcohol
- ☑ Take your own food
- ☑ Be the host
- ☑ Rethink the emphasis on food at holiday time
- ☑ Keep moving
- ☑ Avoid stores the day after a holiday
- ☑ Fast when you can
- ☑ Stay far away from the party table
- ☑ Communicate, don't consume

HANDLING A CRISIS

When we are faced with a crisis, we often need fast food fast. We need energy and comfort, often in great quantities, and always immediately. If we are emotional overeaters, emergencies can send us to the cookie jar as fast as a fire truck to a fire.

So, how do we keep our paleo heads on when all around us are losing theirs? Crises, by their very nature, are not normal events. They are extraordinary, and they require extraordinary responses. How do we keep to our normal paleo eating habits in the middle of a maelstrom?

MAKE A COMMITMENT TO HEALTHY EATING

There's an argument to be had that, in the eye of the storm, sweets and carbs have their place. You're operating for many hours flat-out and without rest. Everyone is relying on you, and you have to be "on." Cue the sugar, fat, carbs, and caffeine to provide you with that energy. And maybe it works for a short while, but if it goes on for more than a few hours – a few days, weeks, or months – this behavior will stick you down a hole in terms of your health and energy, and you can't solve any problems from down there. Make a commitment to eat healthily during this time and make it a priority. Resolve to establish new, or adapt existing, paleo strategies to your new situation that will sustain you for the longer term, especially if your crisis morphs into a major life change. Jam a stick in the carb-fuelled hamster wheel spokes. Stop it from turning before it gets a grip. You need to maintain your energy and your mood. Your ability to manage the crisis may depend on it.

DON'T BEAT YOURSELF UP

If you do find yourself turning to non-paleo foods to get you through, give yourself a break. It happened; it's over. Tomorrow is a new day. You have enough to worry about.

PALEO SECRET #7: SELFISH IS SELFLESS. CONCENTRATE ON YOUR OWN HEALTH BEFORE YOU ATTEMPT TO HELP ANYONE ELSE WITH THEIRS. LEAD BY EXAMPLE. GET YOUR OWN SKILLS DOWN. ISOLATE YOURSELF FROM NEGATIVITY. FOCUS ON YOU.

START PLANNING YOUR PALEO MEALS AS SOON AS POSSIBLE

Staying healthy during a crisis is essential. Everything comes crumbling down if your health and energy become compromised by an unhealthy diet. Your health is the basis that underpins everything else you do, so make sticking to your eating plan a priority, especially if your crisis is going to last a while.

EAT THE SAME MEALS OVER AND OVER

There is nothing wrong in doing this. Thinking about what to eat has to be half the burden of making meals, in my opinion. Take the energy required to think out of the equation and put it to use working on something else more critical – I'm sure your brain is working at five hundred miles a minute as it is. Simply identify a few easy-to-make, simple dishes. Batch-cook them if you can, and eat them over and over. I got a thing for salads with greens, olives, anchovies, bacon, and eggs when I had a recent crisis. I ate them every day for dinner. There was no cooking except for hard-boiling eggs and frying bacon, which I did in batches. Easy.

DRINK WATER

Avoid the caffeine, even though it might keep you going and going. Keep yourself hydrated – make it a routine to drink your water on an hourly basis if you like. Find something that will prompt you – set a timer, drink on the hour or at every stop light, or every time you start a new chapter of your book, as you sit at your loved one's bedside. Water contains nutrients in the form of minerals that you need and acts as an essential carrier/transporter of other nutrients around the body. It's not as important to eat – you can always fast – but water, that's what you need.

FIND A STRESS-BUSTING ROUTINE

Make it easy, enjoyable, and light. Buy the latest book from your favorite author and read a chapter every night. Meditate. Walk. Take detox baths by adding a cup of Epsom salts, or apple cider vinegar, or baking soda to your bath water. These baths are particularly good if you find you can't concentrate or your mind is spinning. Incorporate your stress-busting routine into every day; make it a priority and do it without fail. Don't skip it; consider it a luxury or an indulgence. It is important for your physical and mental well-being and essential to your ability to deal with the demands placed on you. Extreme self-care under these conditions is vital.

FEEL THE EMOTION BEHIND THE CRISIS

If you don't, you may need to gorge on sweets to calm yourself, so it is important to give yourself time to feel the emotions that accompany your charged situation. And that's true even if your experience is a positive one such as the birth of a baby – there are gains and losses in every situation, those that appear bad and also those that are good. Take yourself away from the frenzy, write in a journal, go for a walk, curl up in bed, or talk to a friend. Anything to slow down and get to the heart of the issue, instead of frantically sorting things out, organizing people, and doing "stuff".

KEEP SMALL ROUTINES IN PLACE

Routines ground us when there is craziness going on all around. Make your routines light and easy to accomplish. Lighten those routines you do regularly but usually more intensely – this isn't the time to start training for a marathon. Focus on just two or three essential ones – planning and executing dinner, a self-care ritual, or a walk around the block, for example. Focus on these.

ACCEPT HELP

Pull in support from those around you – outsource essential activities wherever possible. *Do not* decline offers of help; by accepting, you are giving others the opportunity to feel good about themselves, it is a travesty to both you and them not to. You are turning down a win-win situation if you do. If people offer to provide meals, state that you eat meat and veg, and berries for dessert – simple, clear instructions. When people ask you what you need, and you can't think of anything, write their name and number down. As items that you can delegate occur to you, write them down, too. Call those people who've offered to help as your needs become apparent over the coming days. If you can't function, have someone (maybe two – this is a tough job) who can field interference and offers of help for you. A community will come forth and help you – if you let it.

BE PRESENT

Sounds a bit "woo", doesn't it? But it really means to concentrate on what you are doing right here, right now. Don't let your mind wander off; don't think about what you have to do next or for the rest of the day. Just focus on what you are doing in the present moment, however mundane it is. Whether you're cleaning your teeth, driving to the hospital, or answering email, just focus on that, just that. Appreciate the ordinary – it will slow you down and calm you, and really, it's the only way to appreciate life, crisis or none.

CREATE SOMETHING

Anything. Use it as a way to process your emotions. Paint, write, scrapbook, or undertake a DIY project – whatever appeals to you. Plan it, focus on it, and complete it. Like your routines, make this light and easy to do. Think about what you enjoyed as a child and do that. Get a paint-by-numbers kit or knit a scarf. Organize your books into alphabetical order. It doesn't have to be meaningful to anyone else except you. Make it something that gives you a feeling of satisfaction and accomplishment once you're done.

Handling a Crisis Checklist

- ☑ Make a commitment to healthy eating
- ☑ Don't beat yourself up
- ☑ Start planning your paleo meals ASAP
- ☑ Eat the same meals over and over
- ☑ Drink water
- ☑ Find a stress-busting routine
- ☑ Feel the emotion behind the crisis
- ☑ Keep small routines in place
- ☑ Accept help
- ☑ Be present
- ☑ Create something

CLIMBING BACK ON THE PALEO WAGON

We've all done it: cheated; indulged; fallen off the wagon; splurged – whatever you want to call it, it happens. Some follow a plan for indulging, but many are inexperienced and wonder how they came to find themselves in the dust and dirt, banged up from rocks. They shake their heads with frustration and bewilderment as they brush themselves down and contemplate climbing back up to resume the journey.

There are two ways to do it – the hard reboot or the softer reintroduction. I consider myself a master of this type of situation and apply different techniques depending on the circumstances. Let's look at them.

THE HARD REBOOT

This is when you stop yourself in your tracks, skidding quite often, but stop you do. You decide there and then that enough is enough, that one minute more is too long. Kind of like when you're a mom, and you get fed up with your family taking advantage of you, and you go on strike for the evening. Or your boyfriend is bothering you, and suddenly you're done with him, and you don't look back.

It might seem like a sudden change of direction (or even a personality transplant), but most likely, you've been feeling uncomfortable with the state of things for a while and putting up with it. Same goes for your food choices. If you choose the hard reboot, consider these strategies:

MAKE A DATE

The trick with this is to draw a line in the sand beyond which you are back to your paleo plan. Set a date and a time in the future – it could be the next minute, tomorrow, or the moment you step in the house, but when that moment is reached, you're onto the next phase. This works particularly well when you are in a different geographical location. Maybe you've been away visiting family for Thanksgiving or on vacation. Make it a point that the moment you get home, you're back to paleo. When I travel, if I've strayed, I consider the moment the plane wheels hit the home tarmac to be my line in the sand, and from then on I'm back to my usual 98 percent paleo eating plan.

BUILD ANTICIPATION

If you tend to draw these firm boundaries, then have a hard time keeping to them, put them off to a future date. The key thing here is to make a *firm* date for when you'll resume paleo. It shouldn't be too far into the future – certainly within a month – but sometimes the brain needs time to get ready. It has to go through an adjustment, do some planning, or just sit in anticipation. Use this time to make practical plans – collect recipes, make up meal plans, buy some ingredients, and get rid of non-paleo food you don't want hanging around. And when that date comes, you're off, determined, no looking back – the wheels are back on and well-greased, and they're running smoothly.

GO!

The first day of the month, beginning of the week, or the start of the day – anything that implies a fresh start is a good time. It can be whenever you want. You decide.

A GRADUAL TRANSITION

This is when you gradually drop non-paleo items from your diet on a regular basis as a way to gently transition back into paleo. It can be done as part of the anticipation process I describe above, or it can be a process in and of itself as you slowly get back to being more and more paleo over time.

DROP ONE ITEM A DAY

Consider where you are now with your non-paleo eating and resolve to lower the amount every day. I have a friend who is a disaster around chocolate after Halloween. She can't stop eating it. The only way she can do it is if she starts to slowly cut down the number of mini-size candies she eats each day. She does it over a week or so.

SET YOURSELF MINI-CHALLENGES

Doing daily mini-challenges can really help with motivation and confidence if you feel you've lost your way. As you get back on the wagon, these are good tactics to use to tone up your food choice muscles that may have gotten a little weak recently. For example, set yourself a goal to drink a green smoothie or a cup of homemade chicken stock, or to make one meal that day entirely paleo, or to toss out five non-paleo items from your pantry. Come up with your own ideas that are easy to do, and that will get you back on your paleo way.

REPLACE NON-PALEO FOOD WITH THE PALEO VARIETY

As you gradually resume your place in the driving seat of your paleo wagon, get rid of your non-paleo food in whichever is your preferred fashion – throw it away, give it away, donate it, or eat it up. The most important thing is to not replace it when you've disposed of it.

KEEP ON UNTIL YOU REACH YOUR DESIRED VERSION OF PALEO

Whether you follow the 80/20 rule, eat dairy or not, follow a version of paleo that involves restricting certain foods due to sensitivities, or some other personal variation, persistence always leads to progress, which leads to paleo. Just keep at it, and over time you will again reach or even exceed your previous "clean."

Climbing Back on the Paleo Wagon Checklist

☑ **The Hard Reboot**

☑ **Make a date**

☑ **Build anticipation**

☑ **Go!**

☑ **The Gradual Transition**

☑ **Drop one item a day**

☑ **Set yourself mini-challenges**

☑ **Replace non-paleo food with the paleo variety**

☑ **Keep on until you reach your desired version of paleo**

NOTES

(BECAUSE YOU CAN LEARN EVERYTHING
YOU NEED TO KNOW.)

SECTION FIVE:
INTERACTING IN A NON-PALEO WORLD

HANDLING THE SKEPTICS

Oof. I know. It's tough.

Tough to keep your mouth zipped. Tough to smile sweetly and absorb the negativity. Tough to take 'em on and give as good as you get. Tough, whichever way you look at it. Paleo seems to get people going like nothing else. Did vegetarians have to deal with this kind of thing in the beginning?

> NOBODY CAN GO BACK AND START A NEW BEGINNING, BUT ANYONE CAN START TODAY AND MAKE A NEW ENDING.
>
> ~UNKNOWN

Some hard-won advice:

KEEP IT SIMPLE

Don't get into long explanations or complicated language. Keep it to the basics – "meat and veg;" "grain-free;" "I avoid sugar and processed foods." The fewer concepts you explain, the less ammunition you are giving your detractors to hurl back at you and beat you with. The plainer you keep it, the easier it is for the mind to grasp and accept. If someone is cooking for you, but resents the limitations, keeping it simple is helpful and less likely to provoke an irritated reaction.

ROLE PLAY WHAT YOU WILL SAY

Mentally rehearse the situation where your eating comes under scrutiny. Imagine what you will say to your skeptic. Write it down and practice it out loud to yourself in the mirror. Make it no longer than one sentence – your paleo elevator speech.

COME FROM A POSITION OF POWER AND CONFIDENCE

Don't be arrogant, or use a superior tone, and definitely don't knock other ways of eating. But also, don't be deferent, don't apologize, or (and this is common) seek to *justify* your paleo eating. Instead, be calm, serene, and even-handed in your tone. Stick to your short, one-sentence, elevator speech, and say it with confidence. Maintain good eye contact, balance evenly on each foot, chin up, and throat clear.

STONEWALL

Some people delight in an argument. For them, it's entertainment. If that's you too, go right ahead and debate the issues, but if not, do not feed their cause by giving them rocks to throw at you. "Uh-huh," "I see," "That's interesting" work well. Breaking eye contact at the same time and leaving pauses unfilled help too. And, of course, you can always change the subject. If none of these ideas work, you can . . .

DISENGAGE

Walk away if someone wants to get into it with you (they'll call it "a discussion" to maintain the higher moral ground). Remember the great parenting advice: "You don't have to attend every argument you're invited to." Works great for paleo skeptics (and many other situations, too).

KEEP CALM AND CARRY ON

Put a defensive, invisible wall around yourself and appear impervious to stares, looks and comments. Act as normal, including serving and eating your paleo food. And keep an eye on the motivation behind the questions that are posed to you. Often they are well-intentioned, even if it feels irritating. In these cases, a gentle response is more appropriate. Generally speaking, "less is more" in these types of situations.

> YOU DON'T HAVE TO ATTEND EVERY ARGUMENT YOU'RE INVITED TO.
>
> ~JAMES LEHMAN

AVOID YOUR NEMESIS

If you enter a room and someone is there who is likely to step over your boundaries, there is no reason to walk up to them and make conversation. Keep a watch out for them and put distance between the two of you. Once you have practiced your defensive strategies for situations like this, you can take a different tack, but until you have inner power cemented, avoidance is a valid strategy.

TELL THEM WHAT YOU REALLY THINK

You can use this strategy if you like. It's your life; they're your relationships. And it can get utterly oppressive to have such judgment directed at you frequently. However, consider each situation on its own merits before you act. Are you annoyed at this situation in particular, or because of a general feeling of frustration you've felt at past attacks? Or of some other kind of stress? Just saying "no" to Grandma's special apple pie can lead to major anxiety in the early days for some people. If your strong feelings in this situation are the result of some other stress or a buildup, deal with that separately and appropriately. Don't lump all the stress into one and lash out at some unsuspecting person whose innocent question has perhaps tipped you over the edge. Your non-paleo relationships will thank you.

BE A CONSUMMATE LEADER

It takes time and effort to stick to paleo in a non-paleo world. If all your friends are paleo, you have it made. But the rest of us are swimming upstream, and that requires a lot of effort in the beginning. If you work it, though, you can do it. Aspire to be a leader. Really practice your paleo strategies. Get great at living paleo, and the confidence you gain will take you through many challenging non-paleo situations. Your skeptics will simply fall away.

BE A GREAT ROLE MODEL AND GET RESULTS

No words speak louder, and no strategies are more effective.

Handling the Skeptics Checklist

- ☑ Keep it simple
- ☑ Role play what you will say
- ☑ Come from a position of power and confidence
- ☑ Stonewall
- ☑ Disengage
- ☑ Keep calm and carry on
- ☑ Avoid your nemesis
- ☑ Tell them what you really think
- ☑ Be a consummate leader
- ☑ Be a great role model and get results

CONVERTING THOSE AROUND YOU

Can you really convert others to paleo? Is it possible? Can you coerce, force, or manipulate non-paleos to turn to paleo? The answer is, no. You can't. And you don't want to. It's their life and they are their choices. You can only watch their lives unfold, and sometimes that's painful.

You can, however, make it more likely that they will take an interest in what you're doing to the point of giving it a go themselves. And, of course, you can do the opposite and, by your approach, make it less likely they will hear you out and take the lessons on board.

I don't have any particular insight into other people's minds, but I was able to set the stage for my husband to jump the non-paleo ship; I built the gangplank, if you will. He did the walking, though, and took the risk to dive in. I was there giving him the tools and encouraging him. It's a subtle process . . .

FOCUS ON YOU

Explicitly trying to convert someone won't work. It will create distance and cause an enormous amount of frustration. So, focus on *your* journey – analyze your food choices, learn more and more about paleo, and undertake your own n=1 experiments. Turn your attention to you and don't worry about what anyone else is saying or doing, even if they live in your home.

BE A GREAT ROLE MODEL

When others see that you have lost weight, and are more energetic or happier, they will ask you what you're doing. Invited conversation is always more productive, and minds will be open. So, model for others the change and let them come to you.

KEEP QUIET

Don't explain. Don't complain. Don't apologize. Just quietly go about your thing. The less said, the better.

DON'T REMOVE, REPLACE

If you are cooking for non-paleo folks and want to make their meals more paleo, replace a non-paleo item, don't simply remove it. For instance, instead of simply serving a burger without a bun, add an egg to the top of the burger. Make sweet potato mash to replace the regular potato variety. Or make a paleo crust for a pot pie. Replacing an item with a paleo alternative feels less like deprivation, and your family are less likely to focus on what they've just "lost."

MAKE CHANGES SLOWLY

Evolution didn't happen overnight, and transitioning others

to paleo will take time, too. Be patient. Make small, almost imperceptible changes, and don't rush people. They'll push back if you do, and you'll expend a lot of energy getting nowhere. Paleolithic man didn't use energy unwisely, and neither should you. Non-paleo family members have a lot on their plate: they are trying to live their normal life, live alongside a new person (that would be you) and to understand this "weird paleo thing." Give them time to adjust.

BE PREPARED

Don't drive your family mad with your talk of all things paleo. Keep quiet and carry on. But do be prepared if they show a spark of interest. Have materials on hand that they might relate to. Have some ideas for activities they might enjoy, such as paleo books, TV programs, or classes. Overweight spouses might respond to success stories, kids to animal-tracking workshops, and an enthusiastic foodie might appreciate perusing a paleo cookery book. Have them in your back pocket and bring them out when the opportunity arises.

LET OTHERS BE

Accept that you can't change other people. Only they can do that. So, leave them alone. It's hard to be helpless in the face of someone else's struggle; I know that, but the only option is to be the best paleo advocate you can and hope that the someone you love will join you at some point.

Converting Those Around You Checklist

- ☑ Focus on you
- ☑ Be a great role model
- ☑ Keep quiet
- ☑ Don't remove, replace
- ☑ Make changes slowly
- ☑ Be prepared
- ☑ Let others be

LIVING WITH NON-PALEO PEEPS

This is one of the most challenging aspects of being paleo: how to live alongside loved ones (and sometimes not-so-loved ones!) who don't share your eating profile. When it's a spouse, it attaches a whole new level of complexity to marital relations. If it's someone more distant, but with whom you share physical proximity, such as a roommate or co-worker, it can be equally as challenging.

In order to avoid being driven insane *and* keep yourself paleo, here are some suggestions.

CONTROL WHAT YOU CAN, AND ACCEPT THE REST

You can't control other people – their life is their life, their choices are their choices, and the results of those choices are their results. Instead, set boundaries – what's yours is yours, and what's mine is mine, and let them carry on their merry way while you embark on your paleo path. Just make sure that you find some aspects of life that you share together so you stay connected.

RESPECT THE TRANSITION

We all have to go through transitions. We may embark on our paleo way suddenly or gradually, but whichever way we do it, our family members are living with a person who is thinking and doing differently. We need to understand that our actions affect them, and that they will likely change in response to your change, in some way and to a certain extent. They may resist the changes you are making in order to maintain the status quo; it isn't their choice to change, after all. So, we need to be patient with them. They may embark on a number of strategies to announce their resistance as they seek to deal with the changes you are making. They may cook non-paleo food, bring it home, and encourage you to eat it, or want to spend some time with you just as you're going to the gym, etc. We need to understand that it will take time for them to adjust to this new person – you. When this happens, put one foot in front of the other and use all the strategies in this book to help you keep on the straight and narrow.

ACCEPT THEIR TRANSITION MAY NEVER HAPPEN

Your housemates may never come around to your way of eating, despite all your efforts. And that's okay. Focus on you, on your changes, and on your health. You may lead someone to paleo by your results, but fretting, nagging, and manipulating are tactics sure to fail. Do your best, but accept someone else is on their own trajectory.

EXPECT RESPECT

You have a right to eat as you choose and to move as you choose. You don't deserve to be derided for your choices. If you are arguing over food, or your decisions are being ridiculed or undermined, despite clear communication, you have bigger problems than differences over your respective food choices, so get those taken care of. Don't let paleo be your battleground in a bigger war.

MOVE SLOWLY AND OFTEN

> IF YOU WANT TO CREATE HEALTH, WEALTH OR HAVE ANY OTHER KIND OF SUCCESS, YOU HAVE TO BE A WARRIOR.
>
> ~UNKNOWN

Making a radical change is challenging and will bring about behavior that is counter productive as those around you resist the changes you are making. Focus on progress, not perfection. And focus on making progress from the point you are at now, even if that simply means going to a better-quality fast-food restaurant! You can quietly drop a few non-paleo food items from your shopping list or paleo-ize just a meal a week. Simply make one change, then another, and then another. Slowly.

SET LIMITS

Don't eat non-paleo food brought for you by a spouse or co-worker once you've explained one time about your food boundaries. Don't agree to go to restaurants that will sabotage your goals or otherwise do things that don't fit in with your paleo plan. If you do, you will send mixed messages to the people around you.

Instead, discuss what you will eat and accept. Show that you're not unreasonable, but also be assertive and confident in your choices. Others will respect you and your decisions more as a result. Don't be afraid to say, "No, thank you," or, "No, not now, thank you."

ASK FOR WHAT YOU WANT

So many of our eating patterns and choices are ingrained and unconscious that sometimes we have to be explicit if we are to have our spouse and family support us. Ask that the leftover cookies not be brought home from the office. Ask that your co-worker put her bowl of M&Ms out of arm's reach. Ask that your spouse not take the kids for bagels on Sunday morning. Notice what is happening and ask for change.

AVOID ENABLING

Carefully observe your own behavior to see if you are unconsciously encouraging your family to eat unhealthy food. Are you picking up their favorite cupcakes at the store? Do you take them out for ice cream several times a week because it's summer, and that's what you do in the summer? Are you saying, "Yes" when they ask for cereal at the store? Often these practices are unconscious, and sometimes they are driven by guilt. Catch yourself making these types of decisions and decide if they are appropriate.

NEGOTIATE

Come up with a plan that all parties can be happy with. If your co-worker insists on placing a candy bowl between her desk and yours, perhaps she can bring in some candy that she enjoys, but that you find easy to resist. Your spouse can stash the cookies he brings home from the office in a place that works for him, but not tell you where they are. Find a compromise that works for all of you.

THANK THE COOK AT EVERY MEAL

It starts here. If there is only one change you make in your family, make this one. Food sustains our lives, and we need to appreciate it and those who provide the resources to obtain it and who prepare it for our consumption. Make sure adults in the family set the example of giving thanks for the preparation of the meal – whatever has been cooked. Respect is essential; once that is gone, relationships get very, very difficult.

DON'T BE A SHORT-ORDER COOK

You don't have to provide one meal for your family and another for yourself. That will just cause resentment and burnout – in you. Make enough paleo food for everyone and encourage them to enjoy it. If your mealmates prefer to eat non-paleo, give them the responsibility to provide it. Don't enable them by buying it for them. Don't cook it. You could even refuse to drive home with it in your car! If they want it, they need to get it. You can choose not to support their food choices in this way.

GATHER A SUPPORT NETWORK

I say this over and over – make paleo normal for you. Educate yourself, and have a place you can get support when you're wavering. This is particularly true if you have little understanding at

PALEO SECRET #8: MANY BABY STEPS TAKE YOU JUST AS FAR AS A FEW LONG STRIDES. WE NEED TO BE CAREFUL WITH OUR BODIES. AGAIN, SLOW DOWN . . . RELAX . . . BREATHE. THERE IS ENOUGH TIME.

home. Find an outside source to help you, especially while you're learning to protect yourself from the pull of our non-paleo culture.

Living With Non-Paleo Peeps Checklist

- ☑ **Control what you can, and accept the rest**
- ☑ **Respect the transition**
- ☑ **Accept their transition may never happen**
- ☑ **Expect respect**
- ☑ **Move slowly and often**
- ☑ **Set limits**
- ☑ **Ask for what you want**
- ☑ **Avoid enabling**
- ☑ **Negotiate**
- ☑ **Thank the cook at every meal**
- ☑ **Don't be a short-order cook**
- ☑ **Gather a support network**

INVOLVING CHILDREN

Wonderful things can happen when children are involved in paleo. Behavior, health, and grades can all improve. The more you involve children in the decision-making and process related to food preparation, the more receptive they become, and the more paleo benefits ensue.

EXPLAIN PALEO TO THEM

Explain in a matter-of-fact way how and why you eat the way you do. Make the connection between any tummy aches or other conditions they complain of, if you suspect food as the cause. Use the great paleo books for kids – *Paleo Pals: Jimmy and the Carrot Rocketship,* by Sarah Fragoso, and *Eat Like a Dinosaur,* by Paleo Parents. Read them to your kids over and over. Get a bookstand and display them in your home like they do in libraries. I wish these books had been around when my kids were younger. How could you not want them in your house?

TAKE THEM SHOPPING

Simply by taking them to a good grocery store or farmers' market, your kids will get more insight into meal preparation than the vast majority of children ever see. Many kids only ever experience food after it has been processed or cooked! But if you take them with you to the grocery store, and especially if you talk to them about it as you do so, your kids will experience meat and produce before it ends up cooked on their plate, and they will see that real food doesn't come in packages or boxes. They'll also get to talk to butchers who'll answer their questions. They get to do math and learn about different vegetables. They learn to help mommy and daddy. And this, in turn, will stimulate an interest in the next stage of the process – cooking.

VISIT A RANCH

PALEO SECRET #9: LESS IS MORE. LESS EXERCISE MAKES FOR GREATER RESULTS.

More great things happen here. Search for a ranch that will give you a tour or find one that will let you simply wander around. Many have orchards for fruit picking and picnic areas you can visit. Again, getting the kids back to the source of the food is the crucial thing here. Explore the ranch website with your kids before you visit to give them more context, and go with questions ready.

INVOLVE THEM IN MEAL PREPARATION

All this getting back to dirt will incite the kids to want to cook. Get them involved in meal preparation so they don't get stuck on baking. They can pull out saucepans, pour, stir, and measure. They can then progress on to getting more and more involved, until they are cooking whole meals by themselves. If they can't, or don't like to cook, get them involved in other ways. Have them unload your shopping and put it on the shelves, or check the groceries off your receipt as they are put away. They can lay the table or help wash up. Make it easy for younger kids to lay the table by keeping cutlery in pitchers that are kept on the countertop, and mats stored in child-height drawers or cupboards.

LET THEM CONTRIBUTE TO MEAL PLANS

Kids are more likely to eat food they have been involved with, so let them choose dishes for the family menu each week. Give them choices from a paleo list of alternatives or have them search for a recipe they would like to try.

GROW VEGETABLES

The great thing about getting kids involved in this is that you can go at your own pace. A few seeds or a major vegetable plot – it is your choice. Give each child responsibility for either one part of the process or their own vegetable to tend. When they're ready, have them harvest their crop and choose their recipe. They can even cook the meal themselves, truly giving them a "dirt-to-dinner" experience.

GET THEM OUTSIDE

Once upon a time, no one would have had to say that. Nowadays, parents have to get more specific, and often directly involved to encourage outside play to happen. Limit the computer time, take them out to country parks, and invite friends along if they are resistant. Make it a focus to plan outdoor family time rather than visits to the movies and the like. Sometimes it takes a change of emphasis on the part of the whole family to incorporate these activities. Look for inactive time spent watching television or playing video games, and see if outdoor activities can be put in place instead. See if you can incorporate different types of activity into one – walking to the movie theater, for instance. My family even once watched a play acted in different locations, which required a five-mile hike between scenes!

HAVE A FUN, CREATIVE PALEO HALLOWEEN

There are many, many alternatives to the candy-fest that is Halloween. These range from going to a candy-free party to buybacks where you trade in the junk candy for something of superior quality (or even money!). You can switch the candy out, under the cover of darkness when the kids are asleep, for something more paleo. If you create a whole adventure around it, involve them in the process, and capture their imagination, the kids will love it! Buy used books at thrift stores and create a store in your front room for trade-ins of candy for books. Donate the candy to a local dentist in exchange for a donation and have the kids pack it up. Write up a story of the "Switch Witch" who comes in the night to take it away and read it to your kids. The possibilities are endless with some imagination and preparation.

CREATE A FAMILY CHALLENGE

Decide on a goal and work towards it. Find a "hook" to draw your kids in. My son loves to play baseball, and he wanted more upper-body strength to hit with, so he and my husband started doing pull-ups together. Over the holidays we hold our "12 Hikes of Christmas" that started as training for a school back-packing trip, but now has morphed into an annual activity for the fun of it.

TEACH YOUR KIDS CONFIDENCE

Talk to your kids about making the right choices for themselves irrespective of the choices made by other people. In other words, teach them to say, "no." We do it for street drugs and alcohol, so why not for unhealthy food? Unless you live in a very close-knit, isolated group, your children will be surrounded by other kids who eat differently, who may make fun of their eating or encourage them to eat junk food, so it makes sense to do this now rather than after the fact. Explain how and why you eat like you do and point out the effects food can have. But don't nag. Trust your children to make good choices once they have the tools and information to do so.

Involving Children Checklist

- ☑ **Explain paleo to them**
- ☑ **Take them shopping**
- ☑ **Visit a ranch**
- ☑ **Involve them in meal preparation**
- ☑ **Let them contribute to meal plans**
- ☑ **Grow vegetables**
- ☑ **Get them outside**
- ☑ **Have a fun, creative paleo Halloween**
- ☑ **Create a family challenge**
- ☑ **Teach your kids confidence**

NOTES

(BECAUSE YOU HAVE TO DO THE WORK.)

SECTION SIX:
BUILDING A STRONG PERSONAL PALEO CORE

MOTIVATING YOURSELF WHEN YOU'RE STRUGGLING

It's easy in the beginning – you have tons of enthusiasm and lots of energy. You're seeing great gains from your new way of living. But then you hit a bump, you have a setback, the weight loss stalls, and it gets harder. You realize this is for life, and there's no going back – and you're not sure how you feel about that.

Keeping yourself motivated when you're over the initial enthusiasm is hard, especially if you're surrounded by non-paleo temptation. How can you keep this paleo thing going?

SET A SMALL GOAL

Inertia is a supremely powerful force. Kingdoms, fortunes, and more have been lost through lack of action. The effort to get yourself moving is the hardest to summon, but once you're on a roll, well, you're on a roll. So, set yourself a small goal to overcome the drag of inaction. If you want to lose a 100 lbs, set yourself the goal of five. If you want to revamp your entire family menu, do it one recipe at a time. Just start with a goal that seems very doable.

GET PASSIONATE ABOUT PALEO AND THE POSSIBILITIES

Get super-excited. Read inspiring success stories. Visualize how losing weight will make you feel, and what you'll be able to do. Write a bucket list of things you want to do with your life that greater health will support you in achieving. Sit and daydream about it. Really, really want what paleo can offer.

HOLD YOURSELF BACK FROM GOING ALL-OUT

Struggling can be a sign that we're going too hard, too fast. Sometimes, we do need a break; we are exhausting ourselves. Recognize that, and ease off just a little. Not entirely, and not for long, but just to satisfy slightly whatever that little voice or your body is telling you. Release the tension just slightly.

JUST DO IT

In *The War of Art*, author Steven Pressfield says that we only resist doing those things that cause us to grow as individuals. Recognize procrastination and avoidance as a sign that you are moving in the right direction. Embrace the resistance and do it anyway.

REPLACE NEGATIVE THOUGHTS WITH POSITIVE ONES

Tell yourself, "If (insert person's name here) can do it, so can I." Talk to yourself like you would to your best friend. Be your own coach. Remember to be kind to yourself, especially if you're someone with an over-developed sense of responsibility, or you have a tendency to beat yourself up. And remember, you come from tough stock; you wouldn't be here if your ancestors were anything but.

CONNECT WITH LIKE-MINDED FRIENDS AND STAY ACCOUNTABLE

Go online and find paleo buddies, or, if you know people in real life, call them up. Suggest a meet-up. Hang out with people who are paleo successes and those committed to living the paleo life. Keep checking in with your buddies, your forum, or your blog readers – whoever you've publicly stated your intentions to.

IF YOU ARE GOING TO HAVE A TREAT, ENJOY EVERY FREAKIN' BITE. LOOK AT IT WHEN YOU EAT IT. EAT SLOWLY. DON'T UNCONSCIOUSLY SHOVEL IT INTO YOUR MOUTH. AND DON'T CONSIDER IT "FALLING OFF THE WAGON."

~TARA GRANT

READ INSPIRING STORIES

Read the success stories over and over, if necessary. (Mark's Daily Apple has one every Friday.) Search on "paleo success stories" in Google. Print them out and make up scrapbooks or bookmark them. Refer to them whenever you need to. *The Paleo Miracle: 50 Real Stories of Health Transformation*, is a book entirely devoted to paleo success stories. Make that part of your paleo library.

BUILD SUCCESSES

Celebrate each baby step and add another one. Write them down. Make a list of them and regularly look at what you've written to monitor your progress. Really notice and enjoy the pleasure in achieving your baby steps and larger goals. We don't do enough of this (and I am terribly guilty myself). Savor achieving your goal. Sit back, relax, and reflect for a moment. Don't rush on to the next thing. How does it feel? Good, right?

REWARD YOURSELF REGULARLY

Make a list of appropriate rewards – make some rewards small, such as reading a chapter of your current novel, and others larger, such as maybe a facial or a new exercise toy. As you achieve your goals, reward yourself with items from this list. Tie the size of your reward to the size of your achievement. Make sure your rewards do *not* involve food! You should be rewarding yourself at least once a day. And you may find the satisfaction of reaching your goal is motivation enough – no need for outside help.

REVIEW THE BENEFITS

Go back to the beginning. Make a list of reasons for wanting to be paleo and list the benefits of your doing it well. Review this list at least once a day. Put it in your phone or stick the list on your bathroom mirror. Focus on it to remind yourself and train your brain to understand the reasons for your doing what you do.

Visualize how achieving your goal is going to feel. Consult your list to insert a pause between wanting to succumb and actually doing so. Often, a pause is enough to stop you in your tracks.

SET YOURSELF MINI-CHALLENGES

While you might do these when transitioning back into paleo after a period of indulgence, you can also do them to get yourself re-motivated. Do them to experiment, challenge yourself, tune-up, hold your interest, or start a habit. Focus on things you could (and perhaps should) be doing more of, such as eating more sauerkraut, or set yourself a press-up or kettlebell challenge. Other examples might be no dairy for a day, cook two new recipes during the week, or plan to sleep eight hours a night at least four nights out of five. Make them as light or intense, and as long or short, as you think you can achieve – a month; a week; a day – and mix them up frequently to keep your interest alive.

GET HELP

Hiring a coach can be awesome. We often put this idea off, telling ourselves we can't afford it, but, to be honest, whenever I've gone and hired one (and often I've felt I can't afford it), I've found the payoffs to be huge. The cost has always turned out to be trivial compared to the benefits I've received. So, consider hiring one in the area you need help with. It doesn't have to be a personal trainer, it could be a life coach or a weight-loss coach, or a therapist in cognitive behavioral therapy – someone who can help you achieve your goals and support you through your self-defeating behaviors and slump. Consider them part of your "success team." And if there's a paleo seminar going on in your area, go to it – there's usually a wealth of information to be gleaned, and you'll get to meet like-minded people.

MAKE YOUR GOAL EVEN SMALLER AGAIN, TINY EVEN, ALMOST APPARENTLY POINTLESS

Still can't get motivated? Set a teeny, tiny goal, one you can do practically with your eyes shut. Don't set the expectation that you'll do anything more. Struggling to find the energy to cook a paleo meal? Get out the recipe book. Gone on a non-paleo binge? Make your next *bite* a paleo one. Can't get motivated to work out? Drive to the gym's parking lot. Often times, even though you've set a ridiculously easy goal, you'll find yourself exceeding it – you'll get to the gym parking lot and find yourself walking inside, for example. But even if you don't, repeat the goal the next day, and this time push yourself just a little further – walk inside the building, for example, or get out the ingredients for your recipe.

NEVER SKIP MORE THAN TWO DAYS IN A ROW

Two days missed seems to be the dreaded number required to derail a habit. One skipped day is okay, but two days, and the effort required to get back into it on the third day is often more than a lot of us can muster.

BE AWARE OF YOUR URGES TO QUIT AND PLAN TO OVERCOME THEM

Tally your urges to quit throughout a day. Note when they show up and anticipate them. Perhaps you fall foul of the vending machine at 4 p.m. – so, eat something nourishing at 3 p.m. Develop a plan for handling those urges, and write your plan down and action it.

GET THROUGH YOUR LOW POINTS

We all have low points, feelings of failure. Wait for your enthusiasm to come back – it will. Meanwhile, do all the above actions and keep the end game in mind – a healthy, smooth-running body.

WRITE DOWN WHAT YOU'VE DONE RIGHT RECENTLY

You'll surprise yourself. We focus so much on what we do wrong that we completely overlook our successes, especially the small, daily ones – walking instead of taking the elevator, the cup of chicken broth we had with our lunch, or the respectful way we asked our co-worker to move her bowl of candy to a location out of arms reach. Instead of beating your own behind, pat yourself on the back.

Motivating Yourself Checklist

- ☑ Set a small goal
- ☑ Get passionate about paleo and the possibilities
- ☑ Hold yourself back from going all-out
- ☑ Just do it
- ☑ Replace negative thoughts with positive ones
- ☑ Connect with like-minded friends and stay accountable
- ☑ Read inspiring stories
- ☑ Build successes
- ☑ Reward yourself regularly
- ☑ Review the benefits
- ☑ Set yourself mini-challenges
- ☑ Get help
- ☑ Make your goal even smaller again, tiny even, almost apparently pointless
- ☑ Never skip more than two days in a row
- ☑ Be aware of your urges to quit and plan to overcome them
- ☑ Get through your low points
- ☑ Write down what you've done right recently

AVOIDING YOUR FAVORITE NON-PALEO TEMPTATIONS

This seems to be one of the hardest challenges of all. How do we resist all those foods that we know, intellectually, are poisonous to us but emotionally support us? The fact that they are readily available can feel like torture.

CLEAR THE HOUSE

This is dependent on the people you live with, but if you can, avoid all temptation in the home. If you have a craving or merely fancy some non-paleo food, but you have to go out and purchase it, oftentimes you'll consider the effort to do so not worth it.

PUT TEMPTATIONS IN INACCESSIBLE/ DIFFICULT-TO-GET-TO PLACES

The harder it is to access, the less likely it is you'll go for it. I suggest high shelves, corners of the garage, freezing the food solid in the freezer. Every barrier you can put between you and eating it will help. If necessary, have those you live with hide their non-paleo treats and not tell you where they are.

LOCK THEM AWAY

Give your non-paleo housemates the key. It is not overkill to go and buy a lock box, if necessary. Do whatever you have to to get your cravings down to a place where your blood sugar has stabilized and you can be more reflective about your choices.

BUY ONE SINGLE PORTION AT A TIME

Or break a larger quantity down and put the spares in a place that's difficult to get to. Note: This may not work for abstainers, who often need to eat their fill until they are satiated.

TAKE DIFFERENT ROUTES AND AVOID CERTAIN PLACES

Prevent your temptations being within easy reach. Avoid passing by your co-worker's candy bowl. Don't work on your laptop in the coffee shop where the pastries will call your name. Drive a different way to work so you don't pass by fast-food restaurants. Become aware of your surroundings and take avoidant action. When I was a young waitress, the chocolate mints given out with the check were stored by the swing door into the kitchen. Many, many times a night I had to pass by that box. And that tortured me. By the end of the evening, I was ready to down a whole case of the things. So, I moved them to a quiet, out-of-the-way place. It wasn't so convenient, but it was a corner of the restaurant I didn't pass much. Problem solved. I wasn't constantly tempted or tortured.

CUT DOWN THE VISUALS

Record your TV shows and skip through the ads. There are way too many restaurant and junk-food commercials shown on TV designed to tempt you. The ads are carefully created to get your salivary glands going, and they'll succeed – you'll soon be reaching for the munchies. Ignore them by never watching shows live and fast forwarding through the commercials. Or press "mute" and read a book.

VISUALIZE THE DAMAGE THESE FOODS ARE DOING

When someone on my Facebook page said that wheat turns into glue inside us, it had a major effect on me. Reading about the damage sugar does to our bodies helps with resisting that, too. Create an image or a metaphor for the effect these foods have on you and remind yourself when you're tempted.

TEST YOUR BLOOD SUGAR

If you have access to a blood-sugar monitor, check your blood-sugar levels in the morning before you've eaten anything and then again after you've eaten a piece of cake or a cookie. Intellectually, we may understand that unhealthy food is bad for us, but seeing the effect it has on us in black and white (even if we haven't manifested a health problem yet) can deter even the most determined sugar addict.

PREPARE A BATTLE PLAN AND FOLLOW THROUGH

GOOD IDEAS ARE NOT ADOPTED AUTOMATICALLY. THEY MUST BE DRIVEN INTO PRACTICE WITH COURAGEOUS PATIENCE.

~HYMAN RICKOVER

Write your strategies down so that you prepare your own personal manual designed to avoid your trigger foods. For each situation you know is coming up where there will be temptations, sit down and write up a battle plan. Use this book as inspiration and keep it with you. Be the warrior you need to be – anticipate every possibility and plan a response. Then, practice your response. Pin your list up, and put your plans into your phone and on your desk. Review them regularly, and put them into action. Record your progress daily and review on a monthly, six-monthly and annual basis.

CHANGE YOUR LIFE

If you want something badly enough, you'll make sacrifices. You have to. Olympic athletes do, and people who lose a huge amount of weight do. Are **you** willing to? Perhaps you need to do something drastically different – lose those friends who go drinking, decline those invitations, and break up with the boyfriend who supports, enables, and even encourages your unhealthy habits. Go to the gym instead, snuggle up in your paleo oasis, and find some new friends. Do something majorly different, because your body is the only one you have, and it is worthy of sacrifice.

DECIDE IF YOUR BODY NEEDS SOMETHING DIFFERENT

Are you struggling to resist your temptation foods because your body requires some input it isn't receiving? Could you take care of it some other way so that it doesn't demand the glucose injection, the serotonin, or the feeling of fullness. Does it need more protein or (and this is a common one) more fat, or simply more food? Work out what your body is telling you and go meet that need.

MAKE BETTER CHOICES

I have a confession to make: I regularly travel to London, and I would eat chocolate on the return journey. The trip takes place during daylight hours and is preceded by a two-hour drive to the airport and two hours hanging around. All told, it is a sixteen-hour journey home, during which I am awake the entire time. About nine hours into the trip, the flight cabin crew come around with the duty-free cart. On that cart are multiple large bags of my favorite chocolate candy and, bored out of my mind and with another seven hours to go, I would invariably succumb. When I considered how to turn this situation around, I looked at the various options, considering I was at a weak point with my willpower and likely to continue to indulge.

PALEO SECRET #10: LOCK DOWN THE KEYS TO THE SECRETS OF LIFE. PERSISTENCE AND DETERMINATION LED YOU TO THIS POINT AND WILL TAKE YOU FURTHER TO WONDERFUL PLACES IN LIFE IF YOU KEEP GOING. KEEP COURSE-CORRECTING, TESTING, EXPERIMENTING, AND WHEN YOU FIND THE COMBINATION THAT UNLOCKS YOUR SAFE, KEEP IT SECURE SO YOU NEVER LOSE IT AGAIN.

The options I considered were: not flying (not possible); changing the airline (not preferable); and buying something healthier on-board (not possible and, anyway, not likely). I settled on taking dates on board with me. I tend to eat too many dates at one time (I can't control them) so, I don't buy a whole container, I buy just the number I need from the bulk goods aisle the day before I fly. I take them on the flight with me and pull them out when the duty-free cart comes around.

This way my need for a treat is satisfied at that dull, dull point in the trip. When faced with a dilemma like this, go for the lesser evil. It may not be a perfect paleo choice, but if in every situation you make the best one you can, you will find that you'll make better and better choices until the decisions you make are awesome!

CREATE A BETTER LIFE FOR YOURSELF

We reach for our comfort foods when we are depressed, unfulfilled, or uninterested in our lives. If we are continually under-invested in our lives, we need to change that, not eat more. Work out if this is you, and, if it is, what you need to change. As I said in the beginning, don't squander your ancestor's sacrifice. Live the life you were set up for.

Avoiding Temptations Checklist

☑ **Clear the house**

☑ **Put temptations in inaccessible/difficult-to-get-to places**

☑ **Lock them away**

☑ **Buy one single portion at a time**

☑ **Take different routes and avoid certain places**

☑ **Cut down the visuals**

☑ **Visualize the damage these foods are doing**

☑ **Test your blood sugar**

☑ **Prepare a battle plan and follow through**

☑ **Change your life**

☑ **Decide if your body needs something different**

☑ **Make better choices**

☑ **Create a better life for yourself**

NOTES

(BECAUSE RESISTANCE IS A SIGNPOST
POINTING THE WAY YOU NEED TO GO.)

CONCLUSION

Perhaps, right now, you are struggling. And you know it – you're consciously incompetent. Maybe you feel depressed and hopeless at times. You keep falling over and landing with a bump. You're bruised and in pain, and think you're never going to get the hang of this paleo thing. Sugar is your nemesis, and feasts can last days.

Or maybe you've turned the corner, and you see that smooth paleo sailing is possible. It still requires effort, but the cupcakes are rarely speaking to you, you're not reaching for your comfort foods as often, and you're learning to blend your paleo meals and actions into your life. But there's still a way to go.

> MY DOCTOR TOLD ME TO STOP HAVING INTIMATE DINNERS FOR FOUR. UNLESS THERE WERE THREE OTHER PEOPLE.
>
> ~ORSON WELLES

But eventually, with consistent practice and conscious effort, things start to hum. They work. You manage to turn down the pie or resist saying, "yes" to your teenager's plea for frozen pizza for dinner; you make a fish dish instead. You suddenly notice your mind wandering as you walk up that hill, whereas a month ago you had to concentrate agonizingly over every step. Indulgences and treats are spaced farther and farther apart. You're starting to get a grip on the sugar cravings, and your holiday food was a lot healthier this year.

Ultimately, the effort falls away. It won't be necessary. Just like learning to ride a bike or drive a car, living paleo will become effortless. You'll be able to say, "No, thank you" with ease. You'll look at cupcakes, and nothing will stir in you at all. You'll get restless if you haven't done a sprint or a hard walk for a few days.

A process of making small course corrections and steady, incremental progress is the key to mastering paleo; that, and monitoring progress on a month-to-month, then year-to-year basis. Thankfully, we live in times where comfort and food is available at every turn, should we need it. But most of the time we don't, and using common-sense and no-nonsense methods, we can navigate the excess and focus on what's important.

We know we've arrived when we reach stage four of the learning process – the point of unconscious competence – and we suddenly realize we can do this paleo thing without thinking. Now, we've achieved mastery, have integrated the skills, and can look forward. It is an empowering place to be.

RESOURCES

PALEO/NONPALEO INTERNET RESOURCES

For further reading around the subjects discussed in this book, please visit Paleo/NonPaleo. Articles can be found at the following direct links:

4 Mistakes People Make After a Paleo Fail (And What to Do Instead)
http://paleononpaleo.com/paleo-fail-4-mistakes/

56 Concrete Strategies To Guarantee Your Paleo Success
http://paleononpaleo.com/paleo-success-5-strategies/

46 Paleo Tips Anyone Can Do
http://paleononpaleo.com/paleo-tips-anyone/

22 Sure-Fire Tips to Beat Sugar Cravings to a Pulp
http://paleononpaleo.com/sugar-cravings-beat/

9 Sure-Fire Tips to Deflect the Doubters and Achieve Your Paleo Goals
http://paleononpaleo.com/paleo-skeptics-goals-1/

6 Reasons To Eat Junk Food When You Go Paleo
http://paleononpaleo.com/paleo-diet-failure-junk-food/

13 Simple Tips to Paleo Your Way Out of a Crisis
http://paleononpaleo.com/paleo-crisis-overwhelm-tips/

10 Super-Efficient Steps to Hacking Paleo School Lunches
http://paleononpaleo.com/paleo-school-lunches/

150 Quotations To Inspire Struggling Paleo Peeps
http://paleononpaleo.com/paleo-quotations-health-1/

10 Undeniable Paleo Truths You Ignore At Your Peril
http://paleononpaleo.com/paleo-guidelines-truths-peril/

12 Sneaky, Selfish Ways I Converted my Husband to Paleo
http://paleononpaleo.com/paleo-spouse-husband-convert/

How to Turn Down Non-Paleo Food
http://paleononpaleo.com/paleo-refuse-food/

Keep Yourself Paleo Motivated In Less Than a Minute a Day
http://paleononpaleo.com/paleo-motivation/

A Paleo Newbie's Guide to Buying Meat Direct from the Farm
http://paleononpaleo.com/paleo-grass-fed-beef-buy/

8 Dirty Little Paleo Secrets Everyone Needs to Know
http://paleononpaleo.com/paleo-secrets/

RECOMMENDED FURTHER READING

Albert, Rachel
- The Garden of Eating: A Produce Dominated Diet & Cookbook

Cordain, Loren, Ph.D.
- The Paleo Diet: Lose Weight and Get Healthy by Eating the Foods You Were Designed to Eat

Davis, William, M.D.
- Wheat Belly: Lose the Wheat, Lose the Weight, and Find Your Path Back to Health

Deutschman, Alan
- Change or Die: The Three Keys to Change at Work and in Life

Dwyer, Dean
- Make Shi(f)t Happen: Change How You Look by Changing How You Think

Ferris, Tim
- The 4-Hour Workweek: Escape 9-5, Live Anywhere, and Join the New Rich

Fragoso, Sarah
- Everyday Paleo
- Everyday Paleo Family Cookbook: Real Food for Real Life
- Paleo Pals: Jimmy and the Carrot Rocket Ship

Gower, Chrissy
- Paleo Slow Cooking: Gluten Free Recipes Made Simple

Halstead, Pauli
- Primal Cuisine: Cooking for the Paleo Diet

McGonigal, Kelly, Ph.D.
- The Willpower Instinct: How Self-Control Works, Why It Matters, and What You Can Do To Get More of It

Paleo Parents
- Eat Like a Dinosaur: Recipe & Guidebook for Gluten-free Kids

Pressfield, Steven
- The War of Art: Break Through the Blocks and Win Your Inner Creative Battles

Salamar, Joseph, ed.
- The Paleo Miracle: 50 Real Stories of Health Transformation

Sanfilippo, Diane
- Practical Paleo: A Customized Approach to Health and a Whole-Foods Lifestyle

Seib, Jason
- The Paleo Coach: Expert Advice for Extraordinary Health

Shanahan, Catherine, M.D., Shanahan, Luke
- Deep Nutrition: Why Your Genes Need Traditional Food

Sisson, Mark
- The Primal Blueprint: Reprogram Your Genes for Effortless Weight Loss, Vibrant Health, and Boundless Energy
- The Primal Connection: Follow Your Genetic Blueprint to Health and Happiness
- The Primal Blueprint 21-Day Total Body Transformation: A Step-By-Step Gene Reprogramming Action Plan
- The Primal Blueprint 90-Day Journal: A Personal Experiment (n=1)
- The Primal Blueprint Cookbook: Primal, Low Carb, Paleo, Grain-Free, Dairy-Free and Gluten-Free
- Primal Blueprint Quick and Easy Meals: Delicious, Primal-Approved Meals You Can Make In Under 30 Minutes
- Primal Blueprint Healthy Sauces, Dressings and Toppings

Smith, Orleatha

- Cooking Against The Grain: Grain-Free Meals That Are Fast, Freezer-Friendly and Fantastic!

Staley, Bill, & Mason, Hayley

- Make It Paleo: Over 200 Grain Free Recipes For Any Occasion

Wolf, Robb

- The Paleo Solution: The Original Human Diet

ONLINE RESOURCES

PALEO LIFESTYLE BLOGS:

Chris Kresser
http://chriskresser.com

Livin' La Vida Low Carb
http://livinlavidalowcarb.com

Mark's Daily Apple
http://marksdailyapple.com

Paleo 30 Day Challenge
http://paleo30daychallenge.com

Robb Wolf
http://robbwolf.com

The Paleo Mom
http://thepaleomom.com

Wheat Belly
http://wheatbellyblog.com

PALEO RECIPE SITES:

Civilized Caveman Cooking Creations
http://civilizedcavemancooking.com

Everyday Paleo
http://everydaypaleo.com

Level Health and Nutrition
http://lvlhealth.com

Nom Nom Paleo
http://nomnompaleo.com

Paleo Parents
http://paleoparents.com

OTHER USEFUL ONLINE RESOURCES:

Eat Wild
http://eatwild.com
Information and, most importantly, listings of ranches around the U.S. supplying grass-fed meat.

Fitday
http://fitday.com
Free online tool to log food activity and monitor weight loss, food macronutrient profile and exercise.

Local Harvest
http://localharvest.org
Find farmers' markets, family farms, CSA's and other sources of sustainably grown food in your area.

Tropical Traditions
http://tropicaltraditions.com
Retail site where you can buy certified organic virgin coconut oil and many other paleo food items of the highest quality, and often in bulk.

T-Tapp
http://ttapp.com
This DVD exercise program packs a punch and there is no better program for giving results in terms of time and money. For the beginner and intermediate exerciser or as an adjunct to a strength and cardio program, this program is great. This is my go-to workout.

Dean Dwyer

http://deandwyer.com

This smart and sassy lifestyle design blog and podcast evolved from Dean's realization that going paleo, losing weight and gaining health is all part of larger change. He aims to empower you with the tools to remake your life the way you want it.

ACKNOWLEDGEMENTS

I'd like to give heartfelt thanks to my husband, Bernard Golden, for joining me on this paleo journey. His guidance was invaluable, and his support and encouragement were essential. And even his reluctance to go paleo in the beginning taught me a huge amount. Thank you, B!

Thank you to Naomi Niles, Peter Guess and Maggie Vittori for turning my words into a book that is easy on the eye and one that satisfies my incorrigible inner grammar critic.

Anabel Jensen, thank you for your wisdom and your listening ears, the opportunities you've afforded me, and the learning I have gained at your feet. I am truly grateful.

To all the paleo experts out there, I feel your work has given me the key to the secret of life. I can't thank you enough.

To my blog readers and everyone who has contributed to my blog posts, I adore writing for you each week. Thank you for allowing me into your lives. I learn more and more from you all the time.

And lastly, thanks to my kids, Oliver and Sebastian, who have taught me more than I will ever teach them. Keep eating your meat and veggies, boys!

THANKS

Thank you for taking time out of your busy, busy lives to read this book. I hope it's been as enjoyable for you reading it as it has been for me writing it. I sincerely hope the information has given you more ideas and strategies for you to squeeze some more paleo lifestyle into your days and years, and a more vibrant, healthy life to boot.

—Alison Golden

CONNECT

Write to me! I want to hear from you. Tell me your issues. Your problems. Your successes. I would be delighted to connect with you:

- **Blog:** http://paleononpaleo.com
- **Email:** alison@alisongolden.com
- **Facebook:** http://facebook.com/paleononpaleo
- **Twitter:** @alisonjgolden

SEND YOUR PALEO SUCCESS STORIES!

For many a struggling paleo peep, it is hearing the success stories of others that motivates them to dig deep and persist. Write to Alison Golden with your paleo success strategies and stories using the email address below. Include your permission for Alison to publish your tale if you are happy to share it with the world.

Email: alison@alisongolden.com

Or you can reach Alison through her website:
http://paleononpaleo.com/contact

27512731R00124

Made in the USA
Lexington, KY
11 November 2013